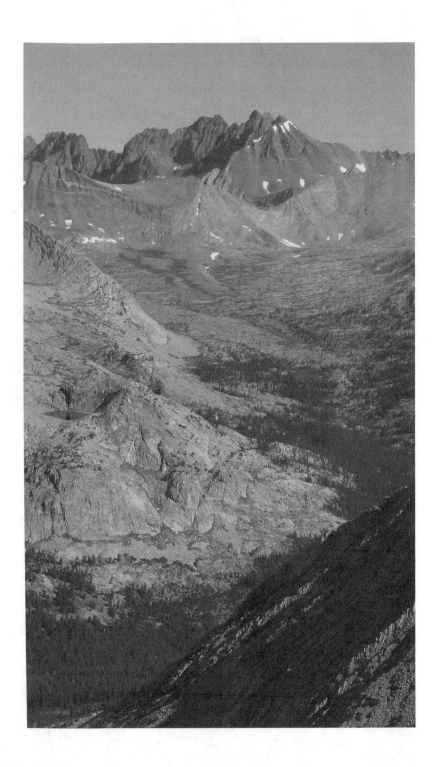

JOHN MUIR TRAIL

The essential guide to hiking America's most famous trail

Elizabeth Wenk
with Kathy Morey

🐏 **WILDERNESS PRESS** ...*on the trail since 1967*

John Muir Trail: The essential guide to hiking America's most famous trail

1st EDITION February 1978
2nd EDITION March 1984
3rd EDITION April 1998
4th EDITION July 2007
5th printing 2011

Front and back cover photos copyright © 2007 by Elizabeth Wenk
Interior photos by Elizabeth Wenk
Topographic maps © 2007 by Tom Harrison Maps. Reproduced with permission.
   Trail maps in this book are from the *John Muir Trail Map-Pack* published by
   Tom Harrison Maps. The 13 waterproof, tear-resistant, four-color, shaded-relief
   topographic maps cover the entire trail from Yosemite Valley to Whitney Portal.
   Tom Harrison Maps publishes shaded-relief topo maps of California's Parks, Forests,
   and Wilderness Areas. All maps are printed on waterproof, tear-resistant plastic with
   mileages, elevations, and UTM grids. Order online at www.tomharrisonmaps.com.

Line maps: Elizabeth Wenk
Book & cover design: Larry B. Van Dyke
Book editor: Eva Dienel
Thanks to David Plotnikoff for helpful comments and advice in preparing this book.

ISBN 978-0-89997-436-1

Manufactured in the United States of America

Published by: **Wilderness Press**
                c/o Keen Communications
                PO Box 43673
                Birmingham, AL 35243
                (800) 443-7227; FAX (205) 326-1012
                www.wildernesspress.com

Visit our website for a complete listing of our books and for ordering information.

Distributed by Publishers Group West

Cover photos: *Front cover, upper left:* Sunrise on the east face of Mt. Whitney;
                  upper right: Banner Peak from Island Pass; *main photo:* Walking through
                  Evolution Basin, with Mt. Mendel and Mt. Darwin behind
                  Back cover, top: Mountain paintbrush growing beside Viriginia Lake;
                  bottom: Walking through Rosemarie Meadow
Frontispiece: The Middle Palisade group and Upper Basin

CONTENTS

ACKNOWLEDGMENTS

Since high school, I have spent every summer exploring the Sierra Nevada, sometimes doing scientific research, but more often just wandering through ever more of the country. I never imagined that my recreation would lead to the opportunity to write a guidebook, especially one on a route as revered as the JMT. I was, of course, thrilled when my friend David Harris (whom I first met while hiking past Silver Lake in 1997) recommended me to Wilderness Press to revise this book. Even though I was three months pregnant, I was not about to turn down this offer and decided I'd simply manage to keep backpacking through the summer.

Revising a book is much easier than starting from scratch, and I thank Tom Winnett and Kathy Morey for their work on the previous text, for it is the foundation of this book. My additions and changes reflect my preferences, including natural history and detours to summits. While I am sad to lose the elegant maps that were in the previous edition, few hikers were still using them. Instead, in this edition we are using the maps from Tom Harrison's excellent *John Muir Trail Map-Pack*. The staff at Wilderness Press, especially Roslyn Bullas and Eva Dienel, have been wonderful to work with. True to their word, they edited my text for clarity, but allowed me to retain my voice as a botanist and geologist.

In this book, in addition to wilderness regulations, I try to express a contemporary wilderness ethic. To this effect, I appreciate suggestions made by many national park and national forest employees. In particular, I thoroughly enjoyed long conversations with many of the backcountry rangers stationed along the JMT corridor in Kings Canyon and Sequoia national parks: George Durkee, Dave Gordon, Kurt Gross, Dario Malengo, Rob Pilewski, and Alison Steiner. Many others answered questions for me and reviewed material I had written, including Mark

Fincher, Cindy Gervasoni, Gregg Fauth, Erika Jostad, and Rachel Mazur. Dr. Robert Derlet, professor of medicine at the University of California, Davis, commented on my text on water quality. Dr. John Wehausen, a bighorn sheep researcher at the White Mountain Research Station in Bishop, helped edit the natural history section. Hikers I met on the trail also contributed to the book's content, telling me what they perceived as shortcomings in the previous edition or other JMT guides, and I thank many unnamed people for their suggestions.

My attachment to all mountainous areas, but especially the Sierra, has been enhanced by having fantastic hiking partners. In particular, my grandfather and father, both geologists, shared their fondness for mountains with me through frequent adventures in the Swiss Alps and the Sierra. Special thanks go to all the friends with whom I have had adventures over the last 15 years, and especially to those whom I persuaded to join me for stretches of the JMT during the summer of 2006: Neela Jacques, Chris Tuffley, and my husband, Douglas Bock. They were remarkably tolerant of hiking with someone who was constantly stopping to take notes and record GPS coordinates. And, of course, I thank little Eleanor for her continuous and good-humored (save a few kicks) companionship on the trail.

—Elizabeth Wenk
Bishop, June 2007

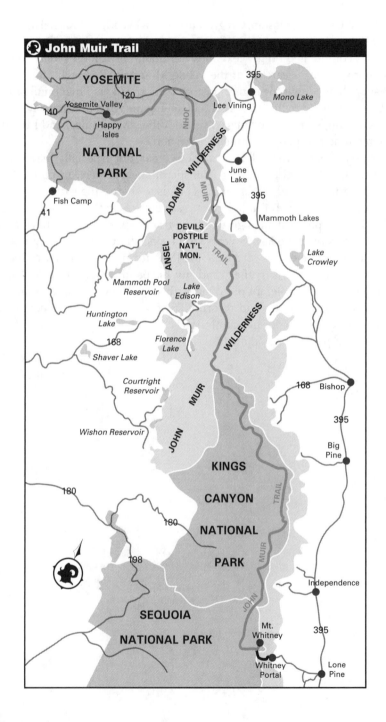

YOSEMITE

120

Yosemite Valley

140

Happy
Isles

NATIONAL

PARK

Fish Camp

41

Lee Vining

395

Mono Lake

JOHN

ADAMS

WILDERNESS

MUIR

June
Lake

395

Mammoth Lakes

DEVILS
POSTPILE
NAT'L
MON.

ANSEL

Lake
Crowley

TRAIL

Mammoth Pool
Reservoir

Lake
Edison

Huntington
Lake

168

Florence
Lake

WILDERNESS

Shaver Lake

Courtright
Reservoir

168   Bishop

MUIR

395

Wishon Reservoir

JOHN

Big
Pine

180

KINGS

CANYON

180

TRAIL

198

NATIONAL

PARK

MUIR

Independence

SEQUOIA

JOHN

NATIONAL PARK

Mt.
Whitney

395

Whitney
Portal

Lone
Pine

INTRODUCTION

The John Muir Trail (or, more simply, the JMT) passes through what many backpackers agree is the finest mountain scenery in the US. Some hikers may give first prize to some other place, but none will deny the great attractiveness of the High Sierra. This is a land of 13,000- and 14,000-foot peaks, of soaring granite cliffs, of lakes by the thousands, of canyons 5000 feet deep. It is a land where trails touch only a tiny portion of the total area, so that by leaving the path, you can find utter solitude. It is a land uncrossed by road for 140 miles as the crow flies, from Sherman Pass in the south to Tioga Pass in the north. And perhaps best of all, it is a land blessed with the mildest, sunniest climate of any major mountain range in the world. Though rain does fall in the summer—as does much snow in the winter—it seldom lasts more than an hour or two, and the sun is out and shining most of the hours of the day. You are, of course, not the only person to have heard of these attractions and will encounter people daily, but the trail really is a thin line through a vast land; with little effort you can always camp on your own if you leave the trail.

This book describes the JMT from its northern terminus at Happy Isles to its southern terminus atop Mt. Whitney, and then to Whitney Portal, the nearest trailhead—nearly 220 miles of magnificent Sierra scenery. For those who prefer to walk south to north, this book also includes a complete description in that direction. The book is aimed at all hikers: Hikers completing the entire JMT in a single trip, as well as those walking a shorter section of the trail; hikers completing the route in 10 days, and those taking a month. As a result, the guide does not include suggested daily itineraries, as each person or group has a different pace, different desires for layover days, lazy afternoons around camp, or detours to nearby peaks or lake basins. Instead, this guide is aimed to provide you with background knowledge and let you design

1

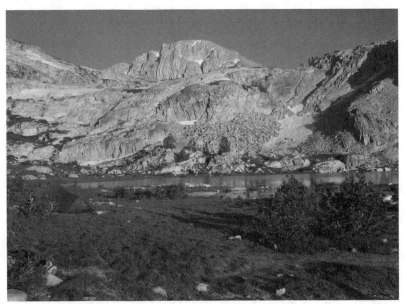

Campsites like this one near Squaw Lake are described in the text and in Appendix C.

your own trip, in advance or as you walk. The book provides information on distances, established camping locations, notable stream crossings, long climbs, especially splendid lakes, detours up worthy peaks, and a bit of natural history to encourage you to gaze at your surroundings. From there, you design the itinerary that best suits you.

The trail description is split into 13 sections, one for each of the river drainages through which the JMT passes. While you are often confined to a single watershed on a shorter walk, part of the glory of the JMT is that you can see how the landscape changes between drainages. Each section begins with a detailed elevation profile of the trail. Marked on the elevation profile are many of the junctions and established campsites you will pass along the trail; this graphical presentation helps you visualize the stretches of trail along which you are likely to find fewer or more camping opportunities.

Also included at the beginning of each trail section is a table listing the major junctions you will pass, as well as some other waypoints. Each entry includes the elevation, UTM coordinates, distance from the previous point, and cumulative distance within that section. The elevations of these junctions and distances between these junctions are also noted in the text using the following notation: [7015′ – 1.5/6.0]. This indicates that you are at an elevation of 7015 feet, you have traveled 1.5 miles since the last junction noted, and you have traveled 6 miles within the trail section.

Following the charts is a written description taking you along the JMT. This covers trail conditions, river crossings, and camping areas, as well as some details of the vegetation communities and geologic features you pass on your hike. (The text is not intended to be read as an adventure story before starting your journey, but rather during breaks as you hike along.) Additional details on many campsites, including their UTM coordinates, are provided in Appendix C. Note that all UTM coordinates given in this book follow the North American datum 1927, as this is the reference system used on all USGS 7.5-minute maps. Many GPS devices and mapping software packages use NAD 1983 as a default, but these can easily convert between the two reference systems.

Finally, one thought to carry, quite literally, on your walk: The nature of the High Sierra changes dramatically from north to south, and often from one mile to the next. With each step, enjoy and absorb where you are, rather than comparing it with where you have been or where you are headed. The grandeur and relief of the southern regions are undeniably striking, but there is no reason to expect (or desire) your entire journey to look like the headwaters of the Kern; if you did, you would spend three weeks sitting atop Bighorn Plateau. Instead, by hiking the length of the High Sierra, you are choosing to embrace the variation in landscape, topography, geology, biology, weather, and more. Could you possibly compare the domes of Tuolumne Meadows, the volcanic landscape near Devils Postpile, the dense stands of mountain hemlocks north of Silver Pass, the lakes of Evolution Basin, the foxtail pines on Bighorn Plateau, or the view from the summit of Mt. Whitney? By the end of your walk, you likely will comment that they are all fantastic and memorable, each in its own way. If a section of the landscape doesn't grab you, watch a nearby stream tumble over boulders, stare at the plants by your feet, follow the sound of the birdcalls to the treetops, or look at the minerals in a rock. These are all part of the continually changing landscape of the magnificent High Sierra.

PLANNING YOUR HIKE

You should not embark on the JMT on impulse. Its length, remoteness, altitude, and continuous ascents and descents mean that you must plan your hike and know what to expect if you are going to enjoy it.

First, you need sufficient experience backpacking to know how your appetite behaves on long hikes, how much your body can take without rebelling, and especially how your emotions react in various backpacking situations. For example, you will have your own typical reactions to solitude (if you go alone), forced togetherness (if you don't go alone), cold, heat, rain, excessive mosquitoes, and injury.

Second, it is helpful to know a bit about backpacking in the Sierra, in order to gauge your expected progress. If this is your first time here, consider the following: The general lack of lousy weather means you can plan to hike for as many hours as your body will take; with few exceptions, the JMT is well-graded with numerous switchbacks easing the long climbs; rocky trails over passes and through some high basins can be hard on your feet, limiting daily mileage; and much of the trail is at high altitude, slowing progress.

Given these parameters, most JMT hikers cover 8 to 12 miles per day, although in this era of ultralight gear (and short vacations), there are also many people ticking off 16 to 20, or more, miles each day. I advocate fewer trail miles per day and a handful of layover days; if you find yourself with extra energy or time, you can always explore a nearby peak (see Appendix E for suggestions) or spend a relaxing afternoon in a picturesque location. To estimate how long the JMT will take you, divide your expected daily mileage into 218.5 to determine the number of days you will be hiking. Add the number of layover days you think you would like to take, and you have the total elapsed days. Using the mileage chart beginning on page 40, the mileage square (Appendix A), and the campsite list (Appendix C), you can pick tentative destinations for each night.

Some hikers prefer to hike the trail in one- or two-week legs, spread over more than one season. This book will help you do that: Appendix B lists accesses to the JMT and how to reach each of the trailheads from the nearest town. Other Wilderness Press publications, including *Sierra North, Sierra South, Kings Canyon National Park,* and *Sequoia National Park,* provide greater detail on these lateral trails.

North to South, or South to North?

South to north is the classic direction to hike the JMT, but rangers estimate that today anywhere from 75 to 90 percent of hikers are headed in the opposite direction, from Yosemite Valley to Mt. Whitney. All hikers I queried were enjoying their chosen direction—and most felt strongly that it was the preferable direction. I took away from my survey that, as expected, everyone hiking the JMT is having a good time and would still be enjoying him or herself if walking in the opposite direction. Nonetheless, I have listed below some reasons why people advocated a given direction of travel:

Some reasons for hiking south to north include:

- The sun is not in your eyes as you walk.
- If your trip is cut short, you have had a chance to see the dramatic, high alpine part of the trail.
- Climbing 6000 feet out of Yosemite Valley in midsummer is miserably hot.
- You are headed the same direction as PCT hikers and can relate to their trail tales.
- It is the classic direction.

Some reasons for hiking north to south include:

- You do not have to put up with the Mt. Whitney permit lottery.
- Your uphills are mostly north-facing and therefore more forested and shadier.
- You are better acclimated by the time you hit the high passes, not to mention Mt. Whitney.
- The scenery just keeps getting more dramatic as you head south.
- Since more people are headed the same direction as you, you will see fewer people.
- This is the direction that the trail was first scouted.

Trail descriptions are provided for both the north-to-south and the south-to-north traveler. Other information, including appendices, is listed from north to south.

When Should You Go?

Several factors may influence your decision about when to hike the JMT, including temperature, snow cover, stream crossings, mosquitoes, flowers, and the number of people on the trail. Each person will, of course, have his or her own opinion on which of these is most important, but despite the differing decisions, just about everyone embarks on the trail sometime between early July and mid-September. It is during these months that you are guaranteed mostly snow-free travel.

Temperatures will be warmest in July and early August. On average, snow cover will be minimal by early July, but there is such enormous year-to-year variation, that there is no normal year, only average snowfall quantities. There is additional information on temperatures and snow cover in the weather section on page 24, including a link to the comprehensive snow pack and precipitation databases maintained by the California Department of Water Resources. Stream levels are strongly correlated with snow cover, such that during late June and early July, on average, stream levels will be very high and crossing can be dangerous. Mosquitoes are likewise unpredictable, but tend to be terrible in early July, tolerable by early August, and nearly absent following the first cold nights in mid-August. The period of the peak flower bloom, unfortunately, lags the mosquitoes by only a week, with the most spectacular displays in mid-July. As the peak flow of people tends to be from mid-July through late August, some hikers choose to begin their trips after Labor Day to experience greater solitude on the trail.

Gear and Supplies

If this will be your longest wilderness trip ever, I recommend that you glance through a how-to-backpack book (such Brian Beffort's *Joy of Backpacking*, also published by Wilderness Press), as well as some online trip reports from other people hiking the JMT. From such information, you should devise your own checklist of essential equipment, including gear you deem necessary for comfort or safety, and possibly extra luxuries that will enhance your trip. If you have purchased new equipment for your trek, be sure to test it before discovering its short-comings on the first day of your long-planned vacation.

Both your gear list and the weight of each item make an enormous difference to your base pack weight—and that is weight that you will carry for 218.5 miles—so think hard about your gear decisions. *Light-weight Backpacking and Camping* (Beartooth Mountain Press 2006), offers plenty of ideas on how to reduce weight. Some of these will make sense to you, others may seem too minimalist, but reading through it does force you to think about what you are planning to pack.

One of the most divisive gear questions is what footwear is appropriate. After many discussions (arguments?) with friends over the correct shoes to wear on a trip, I've come to the conclusion that most options are "correct," but that each person needs to know his or her preference in advance of a long trip. On my most recent hike down the JMT, I wore mountaineering boots, and my husband wore running shoes. We were both very content (and compatible) hikers. His feet and knees would have constantly ached in heavy boots, and I would have twisted my ankles and had sore arches in less sturdy footwear.

Your pack is, of course, made much heavier by the addition of food and water. Most people carry between 1.5 and 2 pounds of food per day. If you were to take 20 days and carry 2 pounds of food per day, your pack would contain 40 pounds of food and likely weigh at least 60 pounds, a pack you are unlikely to enjoy. And, of course, several bear canisters (described next) would be required to accommodate that pile of food.

Few people hike the entire JMT without resupplying. Most hikers arrange to pick up food every five to 10 days. For a few hikers, that may mean a single resupply, usually at Vermilion Resort (87.6 miles from Yosemite Valley and 131.1 miles from Whitney Portal), the Muir Trail Ranch (107.1/111.6), or the Bishop Post Office, accessed via Bishop Pass (135.7/83.0). However, most hikers today pick up three or four food drops, possibly at Tuolumne Meadows (22.9/195.8), and then at the Reds Meadow Resort (or Mammoth Post Office) (58.7/160.0), at either the Vermilion Resort or the Muir Trail Ranch, and at the Independence Post Office, accessed via Kearsarge Pass (177.8/40.9). Details on sending food to these locations and reaching them from the JMT are provided in Appendix B.

In today's era of bear canisters, backpacking food must be compact as well as lightweight. To maximize use of your bear canister, ditch extra packaging and repack any bulky items into small Ziplocs. Many hikers opt for the freeze-dried backpacker foods, but with a little time, and much less money, you can create your own concoctions. Visit a local bulk foods store to find a variety of quick-cooking grains and flavorings. You can likely find several backpacking cuisine books at your local outdoor store.

If you are flying into California and must organize your food for your trip once you arrive here, the stores in Yosemite Valley and Tuolumne Meadows have an amazingly good selection of food for backpacking trips and are competitively priced. Alternatively, the towns of Bishop and Mammoth Lakes have large grocery stores and camping stores. But, foreigners, please take note, full-fat powdered milk is not available in the US; bring your supply with you.

Wilderness Permits

All trailheads accessing the JMT require a wilderness permit and are subjected to quotas. For all Sierra wilderness areas, permits are issued for the trailhead and date at which you begin your hike. This single permit is valid for the entire length of your hike: You do not need to obtain a new permit either when you enter a new jurisdiction or when you exit the JMT to resupply. The one exception to this blanket rule is an oddity regarding Mt. Whitney: The Inyo National Forest website indicates that all parties entering the Mt. Whitney Zone at any time during their trip are subjected to exit quotas (25 people per day). However, agencies other than Inyo National Forest have no mechanism to check the exit quota when issuing permits, and thus ignore it. This regulation may change in the future.

Appendix B lists practical entry points to the JMT and identifies both the agency from which and the trailhead for which you must get a permit. The table on page 9 provides a timetable for permit reservations. This information is subject to change, but the enormous variation between agencies' "when, how, and cost" will probably always exist—don't wait until the last moment to check the agency's website. Throughout the summer season, the Yosemite National Park and Inyo National Forest websites also indicate on what days permits are still available for each trailhead. A word of warning: Quotas for reserved permits fill very fast in summer. Reserve your permit as soon as you know your schedule and, if possible, have alternate, weekday start dates as potential backups. Alternatively, plan to obtain a first-come, first-serve permit the day before. Obtaining permits to begin hikes at Whitney Portal is especially difficult because JMT hikers are competing with everyone wishing to summit Mt. Whitney.

Permit Reservation Information

Agency	When to Reserve	How to Reserve	Cost	Percent of Permits Available for Reservation	First-Come, First-Serve Permit Availability
Yosemite NP	24 weeks in advance	Phone, mail, web	$5 per person	60	Wilderness station opening, day before entry
Inyo NF	6 months in advance	Phone, mail, fax	$5 per person*	60	11 a.m., day before entry, but can fill in request form at 8 a.m.
Whitney Portal (Inyo NF)	February 1, by lottery	Mail	$15 per person	100	Only cancellations available
Sierra NF	1 year in advance	Mail	$5 per person*	60	Wilderness station opening, day before entry
Sequoia/Kings Canyon NP	March 1	Mail, fax	$15 per group	75	1 p.m., day before entry

* $15 per person if exiting at Whitney Portal

Permit Offices

Yosemite National Park Wilderness Permit Office
PO Box 545
Yosemite, CA 95389
209-372-0740 (Monday through Friday, 8:30 a.m. to 4:30 p.m.)
www.nps.gov/archive/yose/wilderness/permits.htm
Note: If you are departing from Happy Isles, you will need a permit for either "Little Yosemite Valley" or "Little Yosemite Valley pass-through."

Inyo National Forest Wilderness Permit Offices
351 Pacu Lane Suite 200
Bishop, CA 93514
760-873-2485 (Wilderness information)
760-873-2483 (Reservation line: October 2 through May 31, Monday through Friday, 8 a.m. to 4 p.m.; June 1 through October 1, daily, 8 a.m. to 4 p.m.)
760-873-2484 (Fax)
www.fs.fed.us/r5/inyo/recreation/wild/index.shtml
Note: If you are departing from Whitney Portal, you will need a permit for the "Mt. Whitney Trail," available only by a lottery held during the month of February. The Eastern Sierra InterAgency

Visitor Center is open in Lone Pine, dispensing both wilderness permits and visitor information.

High Sierra Ranger District (Sierra National Forest)
Attn: Wilderness Permits
PO Box 559
Prather, CA 93651
559-855-5360 (Wilderness information only; not for reservations)
www.fs.fed.us/r5/sierra/recreation/wilderness/index.shtml

Sequoia and Kings Canyon National Parks
Wilderness Permit Reservations
47050 Generals Hwy. #60
Three Rivers, CA 93271
559-565-3766 (Phone)
559-565-4239 (Fax)
www.nps.gov/seki/planyourvisit/wilderness_permits.htm
www.nps.gov/archive/seki/bc_basic/bc_basics.htm

Transportation

This may be California, but it is possible to use public transportation to get to (or from) the Sierra from the San Francisco Bay Area or Los Angeles. Hikers can likewise use public transit to travel between Lone Pine, the closest town to Whitney Portal, and Yosemite Valley. Each of the transit services listed in the table on page 11 provides schedules on their websites; the information in this section covers each service's route and frequency. Much of this information is aimed at hikers arriving at San Francisco International Airport (SFO), Oakland International Airport (OAK), or Los Angeles International Airport (LAX). California residents wishing to use public transit will have to do a bit of their own sleuthing to find the correct connections.

San Francisco Bay Area to the Sierra Nevada: The most direct route from the San Francisco Bay Area (SFO or OAK) to Yosemite is to take BART (see table on page 11 for acronyms) to Richmond, AMTRAK from Richmond to Merced, and a YARTS bus to Yosemite Valley. This combination allows you to travel from the Bay Area to Yosemite Valley in six to seven hours. It is also possible to take AMTRAK to Reno and the Eastern Sierra Transit Authority bus south to the Owens Valley, but this is a longer journey.

Los Angeles to the Sierra Nevada: To reach the eastern Sierra from LAX, you must first take the Antelope Valley Airport Express to Lancaster, a Kern Regional Transit bus to Mojave, a second Kern bus to Ridgecrest, and, finally, the Eastern Sierra Transit Authority bus to the Owens Valley. Fortunately, bus connections allow you make the journey from Los Angeles to Mammoth Lakes, or vice versa, in a long day. Alternatively, one-way car rentals are available between LAX and Ridgecrest, but not to Owens Valley destinations. As the route to/from the Los Angeles area is more convoluted, longer, and more expensive than the one to/from the Bay Area, I recommend flying into San Francisco or Oakland.

Within the Sierra Nevada: The Eastern Sierra Transit Authority system provides transport along the Owens Valley corridor between Lone Pine, Bishop, and Mammoth Lakes, and YARTS provides a daily bus service between Mammoth Lakes and Yosemite Valley. Currently, the bus connections do not allow you to reach Yosemite Valley the same day you leave Bishop or Lone Pine (or vice versa). Instead, you must spend a night in Mammoth Lakes before continuing your journey north or south. Note that the Eastern Sierra Transit Authority site has separate timetables for the bus services within the Owens Valley versus their CREST bus heading longer distances to the north or the south.

Transit Agency Contact Information

Agency	Type	Website	Phone
AMTRAK	Train (+ bus)	www.amtrak.com	800-872-7245
Antelope Valley Airport Express	Bus	www.avairportexpress.com	800-251-2529
BART (Bay Area Rapid Transit)	Commuter Rail	www.bart.gov	510-465-2278
Eastern Sierra Transit Authority (ESTA)	Bus	http://easternsierra transitauthority.com/wb/	800-922-1930
Kern Regional Transit	Bus	www.co.kern.ca.us/roads/ kernregionaltransit.asp	800-323-2396
YARTS (Yosemite Area Regional Transit System)	Bus	www.yarts.com	877-989-2787

Transit Route Information

Route	Agency	Hours	Frequency
SFO or Oakland airport < — > Richmond	BART	1	Every 30 minutes
SFO < — > Embarcadaro (SF Financial Center)	BART	.5	Every 30 minutes
San Francisco Financial Center < — > Emeryville	AMTRAK (bus)	.5	8 times daily
Richmond or Emeryville, CA < — > Merced, CA	AMTRAK	2.5	4 times daily
Richmond or Emeryville, CA < — > Reno, NV	AMTRAK (train + bus)	6	3 times daily
Merced < — > Yosemite Valley	YARTS	3	3-4 times daily
Yosemite Valley < — > Tuolumne Meadows < — > Mammoth Lakes	YARTS	4	Once daily
Bishop < — > Lone Pine	ESTA	1	3 times daily, M-F
Bishop < — > Mammoth Lakes	ESTA	1	2 times daily, M-Sa
Bishop < — > Mammoth Lakes < — > Reno, NV	ESTA	5	Once daily, M, Tu, Th, F
Mammoth Lakes < — > Bishop < — > Lone Pine < — > Ridgecrest	ESTA	4	Once daily, M, W, F
Ridgecrest < — > Mojave	Kern Transit	1.5	3 times daily, M, W, F
Mojave < — > Lancaster (East Kern Express)	Kern Transit	1	7 times daily
Lancaster < — > LAX	Antelope Valley Airport Express	2	7 times daily

Charter Services

In addition to scheduled transportation, the following businesses and people provide private shuttles between trailheads:

Inyo-Mono Transit
PO Box 1357
Bishop, CA 93515
or
703 Airport Road
Bishop, CA 93514
760-872-1901 or 800-922-1930

Kountry Korners Trailhead Shuttle Service
320 Blake Street
Big Pine, CA 93513
760-938-2650 or 877-656-0756
kountryks@aol.com

High Sierra Transportation
Bishop, CA
760-258-6060
www.highsierratransportation.com/

John Pennington
Lone Pine, CA
760-876-4545

Dave Sheldon
Lone Pine, CA
760-876-8232

Additional information is available at the following websites:
www.climber.org/data/shuttles.html
www.whitneyportalstore.com (search message board archives)

Trailhead Logistics

Before you begin (or end) your hike along the JMT, you will need to reach your beginning trailhead and get a good night's sleep. Below is a brief description of how to reach the JMT's endpoints, Yosemite Valley and Whitney Portal, and Tuolumne Meadows, and what camping options exist at each location.

Yosemite Valley

Three California state highways lead from the San Joaquin Valley to Yosemite Valley, highways 120, 140, and 41. All three merge into the one-way loop road that encircles Yosemite Valley. Any amenities you need exist toward the eastern end of Yosemite Valley, either around Yosemite Village or Curry Village. Of particular interest to JMT hikers is the large store in Yosemite Village, which also houses the wilderness permit office and a visitor center. There are a number of restaurants in both Yosemite Village and Curry Village. To the east of Curry Village, on the road to Happy Isles, is the backpacker's parking lot.

Probably most useful, yet difficult to obtain information about, Yosemite Valley has a campground with sites set aside for backpackers for the night before or after their trip. Reservations are neither required

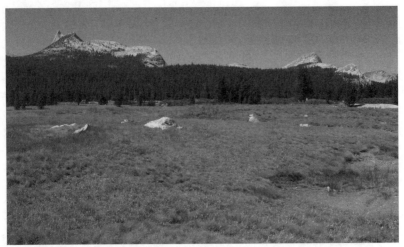

Tuolumne Meadows offers scenic sites and backpacker amenities.

nor available. To find the Yosemite Valley backpacker's campground, proceed to the back of North Pines campground, between sites 331-335, and cross Tenaya Creek on a footbridge. Although you can drive a car to within a few minute's walk of this campsite to unload, you must park your car in the nearby backpacker's parking lot for the night. Throughout the day, a free shuttle bus travels between these locations and to Happy Isles, the starting point for the JMT.

Tuolumne Meadows

Options are more limited than in Yosemite Valley, but Tuolumne Meadows has a small store and the Tuolumne Grill serves hamburger-style fare until 5 p.m. Tuolumne Meadows also has a backpacker's campground, with sites costing $5 per person per night. It can be used for a night by thru-hikers, as well as by hikers, the night before or after their trip. Reservations are neither required nor available. To find it, enter the main campground and head toward the Dana Campfire Circle; the backpacker's campground is due north and clearly marked.

Whitney Portal

Whitney Portal lies east of the town of Lone Pine in the Owens Valley. Take Hwy. 395 to the middle of the town of Lone Pine, turn west onto Whitney Portal Road, and follow it for 13 miles to Whitney Portal. Here, there is a large parking lot, a small cafe and store, and a campground. The 10 non-reservable, walk-in campsites are $8 per person per night, with a one-night limit. In addition, 30 percent of the spots in the main campsite are also first-come, first-serve. Unlike the sites in Yosemite National Park, these are not reserved specially for backpackers, but much of the time you will find a space for the night before or after your hike. Additional accommodation, shopping, and restaurant options are available in Lone Pine.

For more information on campgrounds, including reservable ones in Yosemite and at Whitney Portal, visit the websites for Yosemite National Park (www.nps.gov/archive/yose/trip/camping.htm), Sequoia and Kings Canyon national parks (www.nps.gov/seki/planyourvisit/campgrounds.htm), Inyo National Forest (www.fs.fed.us/r5/inyo/recreation/campgrounds.shtml), Sierra National Forest (www.fs.fed.us/r5/sierra/recreation/camping/index.shtml), and Devils Postpile National Monument (www.nps.gov/depo/planyourvisit/lodging.htm).

Pets and the JMT

Pets are prohibited within the national parks. If you wish to hike with your pet, you are limited to the section of the JMT between Donohue Pass and the Piute Pass junction.

ON THE TRAIL

Seasoned backpackers will tell you that each hiking area has its own idiosyncrasies—both natural conditions and governing body regulations that many people simply haven't thought about until they arrive at the trailhead. Knowing in advance what to expect on the trail will make for a smoother trip. The following sections summarize what you need to keep in mind while backpacking through the High Sierra.

Where to Camp

There are two pieces to the "Where should I camp?" question—the ecological aspect and your personal preference. From an ecological perspective, reinforced by the regulations detailed on your wilderness permit, you should camp 100 feet from the trail or water sources, and never, never camp on vegetation, including meadows. Yosemite National Park, Inyo National Forest, and Sierra National Forest require that you camp 100 feet from water and the trail. In Kings Canyon and Sequoia national parks, it is only recommended that you camp 100 feet from water/trail, but it's required that you camp 25 feet from water/trail. Within these parks, you will indeed pass many obviously used campsites that are not a full 100 feet from water/trail; according to the backcountry rangers, unless areas are clearly posted as "restoration area, no camping," these are legal campsites and it is much better to use an established campsite than to create a new one. The only longer stretches of trail where previously used campsites are not obvious from the trail are those above treeline, where the only campsites are sandy flats among slabs, boulders, or small alpine meadows. If you must camp in such areas, find a patch of sand, or a flat slab, that is 100 feet from water and the trail. Please, never camp on vegetation—it takes years to recover.

After you have taken ecological considerations into account, it's time to think about what sorts of sites you like to camp in. Do you view an alpine landscape as barren and austere or open and free? Does a forest provide you with a sense of protection, is it claustrophobic, or do you simply love looking up at the branches? Is having a beautiful view from your camp or having protection from wind more important? Or maybe you will pick lower-elevation campsites where you can cook dinner faster, where the air is warmer, and where it's legal to build a campfire. If you are traveling in a group, make sure group members are aware of each other's preferences.

Also, think about the following information to help you decide where to camp each night: You will experience more dew the closer you camp to wet meadows or water, especially a bubbling brook; but if you find a campsite that is a short distance into the forest, your gear will be much drier in the morning. Likewise, depressions are cold-air sinks, so the edge of a lake or meadow will be colder than an adjacent knob a few feet higher. Mosquitoes can, and will, be everywhere, but they are most abundant near wet meadows and slow-flowing streams. Higher-elevation campsites, especially those above treeline, have the potential to be windy and colder, but they also have more open views, fewer bugs, and better sunsets and sunrises.

Evening and morning sun are hard to come by on much of the JMT, as you are usually traversing between two large ridges of north-south-trending mountains that block clear views to the east and the west. Still, sections that trend east-west, such as Evolution Valley, have late afternoon sun, and sections of trail that are above treeline, such as the Palisade Lakes, will have much more sun than forested areas deeper in the valleys.

There are at least 200 established campsites along the JMT, giving you ample opportunity to pick your favorite sort of environment most nights. In Appendix C, many of these campsites are identified and described, helping you select the locations and settings that you will enjoy most. Most of the campsites listed are well-used and often dusty. Since you are one of 50 to 100 parties that will use some of these campsites in a given summer, this is unavoidable. If you wish to frequent less-impacted campsites, give yourself a bit of time in the evening to explore farther off-trail for sandy patches amongst slabs or un-vegetated forest floor; but never camp on vegetation just to avoid the dust.

In addition, you will pass through areas with additional camping restrictions. These are usually noted in the text and clearly signed along the trail.

Food Storage and Bears

In the past, hikers have used a variety of methods to keep their food from wild animals such as rodents, bears, and birds. These methods have included sleeping with a food bag, hanging a stuffsack of food off a rock face, stuffing a food bag down a deep crack, and counterbalancing food bags in a tall tree. With the exception of a perfect counterbalance in the perfect tree, these methods are ineffective against black bears, which are very smart and adaptable animals. Since black bears now roam all elevations of the Sierra, especially along the JMT corridor, today's wilderness regulations—and wilderness ethics—dictate that JMT hikers must carry a bear canister. The rangers are pleased to note that there is now more than 95 percent compliance with the regulations, and few hikers are retreating to trailheads after their food disappears in the night. Please keep making the rangers happy.

In Yosemite, bear canisters are required within 7 linear miles of the road and throughout the park above 9600 feet—delineations that include the entire 36 miles the JMT traces through the park. Heading south, bear canisters are likewise mandatory in the Rush Creek drainage and much of the Middle Fork of the San Joaquin River drainage north of Tully Hole.

Within Kings Canyon National Park, if you are not using the bear boxes, bear canisters are required between the Woods Creek crossing and Forester Pass. In both Sequoia and Kings Canyon national parks, bear canisters are required anywhere you cannot find a tree in which you can counterbalance your food 12 feet vertically above the ground and 10 feet horizontally from the trunk of the tree. In effect, you must use a bear canister in all alpine and subalpine areas, where such large trees simply do not exist.

Finally, bear canisters are required between Trail Crest and Whitney Portal. Note that these regulations are likely to expand in the future, so check the Sierra Interagency Black Bear Group website, www.sierrawildbear.gov, for updates.

Over the past few years, the diversity of legal bear canisters has increased and five companies currently produce legal canisters. These are described on the website of the Sierra Interagency Black Bear Group, an organization established to coordinate food-storage policies among all Sierra Nevada national forests and parks. So, no, you don't have to switch canisters as you walk across administrative boundaries. Of the options listed, the Bearikade is very lightweight, but it is also by far the most expensive and is difficult to come by: It is sold and rented only by

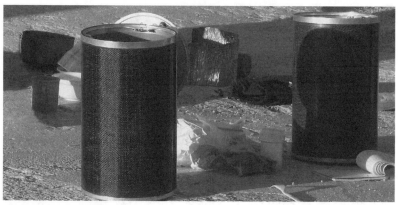

Bearikade bear canisters

the manufacturer: www.wild-ideas.net; 805-693-0550. Many JMT hikers have noted that these canisters can be rented economically. The "Garcia" canisters can be rented from most wilderness permit offices, and if you rent your canister in Yosemite, you can mail it back instead of delivering it in person.

The need to use bear canisters becomes apparent when considering the change in the black bear population in the Sierra over time. Since the early 1980s, black bear populations in California have at least doubled, now numbering between 25,000 and 30,000. Many of those bears live in the Sierra Nevada. In part, this means that ever more bears live at high elevations, elevations where enough natural food simply does not exist—and your food bag looks mighty appealing to them!

Stoves, Campfires, and No-Fire Zones

I strongly advocate the use of stoves over campfires in the backcountry. Using a stove conserves the finite wood supply that is essential for wildlife, plant habitat, and soil replenishment, and it also minimizes the risk of starting a forest fire. If you must build a campfire, keep it small and only build fires within pre-existing campfire rings. In all the wilderness areas you pass through, it is illegal to build new campfire rings.

In addition, many areas along the JMT are closed to wood fires. They are prohibited above 9600 feet in Yosemite, above 10,000 feet in Ansel Adams Wilderness, above 10,000 feet in John Muir Wilderness, above 10,000 feet in the San Joaquin and Kings rivers drainages in Kings Canyon National Park, above 11,200 feet in the Kern River drainage in Sequoia National Park, and at all elevations along the Mt. Whitney Trail. Within the Kern River drainage, wood fires are also prohibited above 10,800 feet in the Wright Creek drainage and within 1200 feet of the following locations: the bear boxes near Tyndall Creek crossing, the Tyndall Frog Ponds, the Wallace Creek crossing, and the Crabtree ranger station. (In each case, these restrictions are relative to the bear box and the adjacent camping area.) As these specifications can change, be sure to study the information you get with your permit on the latest regulations.

Water Purification, Water Quality, and Camp Hygiene

For the last several decades, hikers in the Sierra Nevada have been warned to filter all their water because of potential contamination from the protozoan *Giardia lamblia*, which causes diarrhea and abdominal pain. (Note that symptoms begin one to three weeks following exposure.) As a result, most hikers now use either a filter or iodine tablets or solution to purify their water.

This recommendation remains the status quo, and I certainly do not contest it. However, studies by researchers Robert Rockwell and Robert Derlet (University of California, Davis) indicate not only that the prevalence of giardia in Sierra waters has been far overstated, but also that a number of other, and potentially nastier, microbes have been detected in Sierra waters. Thorough field studies have not yet been conducted on a second protozoan, cryptosporidium, but it is found in lower elevation regions of California subjected to cattle grazing, and it is also expected to be present in areas of the Sierra with high stock and cattle use. Cryptosporidium is of special concern if it spreads to the Sierra because iodine may not be effective in killing it. In addition, disease-causing strains of the bacteria E. coli do exist in Sierra Nevada waters, especially in areas with heavy stock use or cattle grazing. E. coli is killed by any of the purification methods in common use.

Overall, however, few disease-causing microbes have been detected in water not subjected to cattle or pack stock, including areas with moderate hiker use. These studies suggest that many side streams flowing into the JMT may be safe to drink unfiltered—a decision each hiker must make for himself or herself.

A corollary to this information is that some hikers do contract giardia while backpacking, but usually as a result of poor camp hygiene, not consumption of contaminated water. Between 4 and 7 percent of Americans are thought to have giardiasis, most asymptomatically and unknowingly. If you happen to be one of these people, you can easily pass giardia on to your hiking companions through poor camp hygiene. This trend emphasizes the importance of proper waste disposal and food handling. It is essential that all human waste be buried at least 6 inches below the soil surface and at least 100 feet from established campsites, trails, and, most importantly, water. When you pick a "toilet" location, consider not only current water flow, but also that many gullies will carry runoff in spring. All Sierra wilderness areas now require that you pack out your toilet paper. A small Ziploc bag does the trick. Second, if you are a member of a group, make sure your hands are clean before you handle everyone's food.

Backcountry Water

Additional reading on these subjects is available online:
- www.yosemite.org/naturenotes/Giardia.htm
- www.yosemite.org/naturenotes/Derlet Water.htm
- www.yosemite.org/naturenotes/Derlet Yosemite2005.htm

However, even with campers' best intentions, the Mt. Whitney Zone, extending from Crabtree Meadow to near the Lone Pine Lake junction, simply has too many visitors for the "normal" rules to apply; 3000 people camped in the Crabtree and Guitar Lake areas in 2005, generating far more waste than the shallow alpine soils can process. For these same reasons, the toilet on the summit of Mt. Whitney has been removed. As a result, southbound hikers should now pick up a waste bag when they pass the trail junction to the Crabtree camping area and ranger station; these can be deposited in specially marked human waste bins at Whitney Portal. On the Inyo National Forest side, resource managers have determined that the composting toilets that used to exist at Trail Camp and Outpost Camp were overwhelmed, and these were removed in late 2006. Currently, they require that all out-and-back hikers on the Mt. Whitney Trail use waste bags. Northbound JMT hikers are still permitted to bury their waste, as there is no location to drop your filled waste bags once you exit the Whitney Zone. If you are exiting for a resupply within the first week, consider packing your Whitney Zone waste until you are next at a trailhead. These regulations are currently in flux, so please check in at a ranger station to learn the latest policy before you begin your hike.

In addition, to avoid contaminating water, never use soap directly in water, and even when away from water sources, use only the smallest possible quantities of biodegradable soap. This is especially important if frogs are nearby. Research suggests that amphibians, which breathe through their skins, are especially sensitive to the chemicals in either insect repellant or sunscreen. Contaminating the water in which they are living can potentially kill them.

Summer Rangers

A number of summer rangers are stationed along the trail in Sequoia and Kings Canyon national parks (SEKI), and sometimes downstream of the Rush Creek junction, near Waugh Lake, near Thousand Island Lake, and at Sallie Keyes Lakes. In SEKI, there are almost always rangers stationed at McClure Meadow, Le Conte Canyon, Rae Lakes, Charlotte Lake, and Crabtree Meadows. Some summers, you will also find rangers at the Bench Lake and Tyndall Creek ranger stations. The SEKI rangers are on duty from mid-June through late September.

Ranger Pet Peeves

Backcountry rangers know better than anyone how heavy visitor use damages the fragile natural resources in montane and alpine environments. Rangers stationed in different locations have slightly different concerns, but they all identified the following as the dominant sources of resource damage in their patrol areas: creating new campsites, especially on vegetation; inappropriate food storage; inappropriate disposal of human waste, including toilet paper; illegal campfire rings.

You can help stay on their good side by: camping in established sites; using portable bear canisters; making sure your waste is deposited at least 6 inches below ground, and 100 feet from water and trails; packing out your toilet paper; and not building new campfire rings.

Two points deserve special mention. First, rangers can be on patrol for several days at a time, but they always post a note on their station door indicating an estimated date and time of return. If no ranger is present, you may chose to walk to the next ranger station or hike out yourself to report an emergency. Second, remember that rangers have to buy their own food and camping gear, so they, not the government, are the losers if it is taken.

Ranger Station Locations in Sequoia and Kings Canyon National Parks

Ranger Station	Approximate Location	N–S Miles*	S–N Miles	UTM Coordinates (NAD 27)
McClure Meadows (Section 7)	North of the trail, along the stretch of McClure Meadow with many campsites; easily missed when headed south.	16.6	10.1	11S 345384E 4116969N
Le Conte Canyon (Section 8)	Spur trail is just north of the Dusy Basin/Bishop Pass junction.	7.8	13.9	11S 358437E 4106291N
Bench Lake (Section 9)	Across the outlet of the first lake south of the Bench Lake and Taboose Pass junctions.	6.8	3.1	11S 372178E 4091202N
Rae Lakes (Section 10)	Signed spur trail at 11S 375044E 4074834N, toward the northern end of the middle of the three Rae Lakes.	13.0	2.9	11S 375183E 4074633N
Charlotte Lake (Section 11)	Just east of the trail, near the northern end of the lake, 1 mile from the JMT.	2.3	9.5	11S 372906E 4070830N
Tyndall Creek** (Section 12)	Approximately 0.7 mile down the Tyndall Creek Trail.	4.8	18.4	11S 375629E 4054805N
Crabtree Meadow (Section 12)	In trees 0.1 mile to the east of Crabtree Meadow, on the south side of the creek from the JMT.	13.6	9.6	11S 379519E 4047234N

* These mileages indicate the point at which you leave the JMT.
**The Tyndall Creek ranger station is much farther down the Tyndall Creek Trail than is shown on any published map, excepting the maps in this book.

Weather

The southern Sierra Nevada lies between the Central Valley of California and the Great Basin of Nevada. It is primarily influenced by weather from the Pacific Ocean and therefore experiences a Mediterranean climate, with relatively mild, wet winters and warm, dry summers. From November to March, Pacific storms bring abundant snow; during these months, only occasional mountaineers on skis access the JMT. During the spring months, the quantity of precipitation tapers, but the High Sierra is still snow-covered. Depending on the intensity of the winter, the JMT country becomes accessible to hikers between mid-June, in a drought year, and mid- to late-July, in the heavier snow years. The north- and east-facing slopes of the highest passes can retain snowbanks throughout the summer.

Summer moisture is relatively rare, especially compared with the conditions in mountain ranges such as the Rockies or the European Alps. The summer rainfall the Sierra does receive comes up from the south, from remnants of tropical storms originating in the Gulf of California, the southeast Pacific, and even the Gulf of Mexico. Much of the time, this results in a slow buildup of puffy cumulus clouds, which arrive a bit earlier each afternoon and look a bit more menacing. After a few days comes a day or two of afternoon thunderstorms, before the system disappears again. At times, former tropical cyclones may be entrained in southerly airflow, bringing a larger pulse of moisture to the eastern Sierra. This can result in either a rapid buildup of clouds and/ or rain for many hours on end—sometimes even breaking the cardinal rule that "it never rains at night in the Sierra." Any thunderstorm can bring hail to the high passes and peaks at any point in the summer.

Lightning poses the greatest threat to JMT hikers. The clouds can build up very quickly. On many occasions, a cloudless sky in late morning will transform to one with dark rain clouds by mid-afternoon. Should you see dark thunderclouds gathering overhead, do not proceed across passes or through open meadows. Likewise, do not take shelter beneath the only nearby clump of trees, the tallest clump of trees, at the base of a vertical wall, in a cave, or on a saddle; these are locations where you are in the greatest danger of being hit. Instead, choose a location between scattered trees, boulders, or other undulating topography, where you can squat down and vanish beneath the horizon. Be sure to leave your backpack, which undoubtedly contains some metal, a short distance away.

So how does all this translate into the temperatures you are likely to experience on your hike? Daytime temperatures will be pleasantly warm—even hot due to the abundant sunshine. Tuolumne Meadows, at 8600 feet, has highs in the 70s throughout July and August. At night, you are unlikely to experience a frost during July and August, but temperatures will begin to drop rapidly come September. But elevation isn't everything: Nights are colder in Tuolumne Meadows than at Upper Tyndall Creek, nearly 3000 feet higher, because the bowl shape of Tuolumne Meadows makes it a cold-air sink. Data from the automated weather stations at these two locations (and many others) are available at cdec.water.ca.gov/misc/RealPrecip.html.

SIERRA NEVADA HISTORY

In the introduction, I recommended that hikers stop and take in the natural history that abounds in the High Sierra. To aid you in this endeavor, this book is sprinkled liberally with mention of geologic features, plant communities, descriptions of birds that are common in each habitat, and more. In the coming pages are just a few basics on Sierra Nevada natural history. If you wish to learn more about a specific feature or species, there are excellent books dedicated to the subject, which are listed in Appendix H.

Humans and the JMT

In 1884, Theodore Solomons was the first to have the vision of a high-elevation trail, passable by stock, which followed the spine of the Sierra from Yosemite Valley to Kings Canyon. He was only 14. "The idea of a crest-parallel trail through the High Sierra came to me one day while herding my uncle's cattle in an immense, unfenced alfalfa field near Fresno," he wrote in the *Sierra Club Bulletin* in 1940.

After more more than 50 years, Solomons's idea became what we know today as the John Muir Trail, thanks to the efforts of people who explored the Sierra both before and after him. Between Yosemite Valley and Mt. Whitney, features on maps honor John Muir, Josiah Whitney, Theodore Solomons, Joseph Le Conte, Joseph N. Le Conte ("Little Joe"), William Brewer, Clarence King, James Gardiner, Bolton Brown, and Wilbur McClure—to name just a few. Each man helped in the exploration of the High Sierra and the subsequent creation of the John Muir Trail.

The exploration of the High Sierra began with government surveys during the 1860s. State geologist Josiah Whitney was tasked with making "an accurate and complete" geological survey of the state. In

1864, he assembled an impressive team of scientists to spend a summer exploring the High Sierra. His staff included William Brewer, a botanist; Charles Hoffman, an engineer and topographer; Clarence King, a geologist; James Gardiner, a surveyor; and Dick Cotter, an assistant. The party was the first to see many of the sections of the Sierra through which the JMT would later pass: the headwaters of the Kern River, Bubbs Creek, and the country along the South Fork of the San Joaquin River. They also discovered that in the southern Sierra there were two parallel crests, the Great Western Divide and the Sierra Crest, and they determined that the Sierra Crest was over 14,000 feet high.

To survey the landscape, Whitney's team climbed prominent peaks, including Mt. Tyndall and Mt. Brewer. In 1864, King and Cotter made a daredevil crossing of the Great Western and the Kings-Kern divides. King spent years obsessed with reaching the top of Mt. Whitney, and while he did finally make it up the 14,505-foot peak, he was not the first to summit. Unfortunately, this period of state-sponsored exploration was short-lived: Frustrated by the team's focus on exploration and science rather than the discovery of mineral resources, the state discontinued funding in 1865 and later dissolved the survey.

Soon thereafter, Sierra admirers began entering the High Sierra on recreational trips, first exploring the Yosemite high country, and then moving southward. John Muir was one of the first people to head deep into the backcountry, ascending peaks and exploring the country, often on solo "knapsack trips." However, he was a naturalist at heart, more interested in staring at the plants, animals, and rocks than in producing maps of his travels or scouting routes for future parties.

Among the handful of other people venturing into the rugged country during the 1890s and 1900s, three names stand out: Solomons,

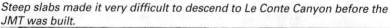

Steep slabs made it very difficult to descend to Le Conte Canyon before the JMT was built.

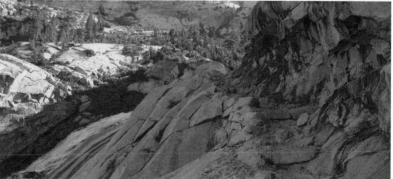

who first envisioned the JMT; "Little Joe" Le Conte, the nephew of Joseph Le Conte; and Bolton Brown. Like Solomons, Le Conte was intent on finding a route, passable by stock, between Yosemite Valley and Kings Canyon, while Brown simply enjoyed long, exploratory mountaineering excursions.

John Muir

John Muir has become a folk hero as the father of the conservation movement. He was the first president of the Sierra Club, filling that role from its inception in 1893 until his death in 1914, and it is said today that more places in California are named in his honor than for any other person. He is even depicted on the California state quarter. However, his contributions to the Sierra were broader, as he published many scientific articles and was also an energetic hiker and mountaineer.

Born into a strict Scottish family in 1838, Muir's admiration for the natural world began as a child. Disheartened by his early jobs in industry, he came to California at age 30, realizing that he wished to spend his life outdoors studying and simply appreciating nature. Following a brief visit the previous year, he arrived in Yosemite Valley in 1869 and spent his first summer as a sheepherder near Tuolumne Meadows. He was immediately entranced by the landscape, its vegetation, and the geologic history.

Muir's name became known for his theories on Sierra glaciation: He was the first to propose that many of the Sierra's landforms, including Yosemite Valley, were created by glacial activity. Although he continued his scientific studies and long treks through the Sierra until his death, his focus soon shifted to the conservation of the mountain landscape. His talks, publications, and interactions with endless visitors to the Valley established the concept of public lands and conservation in the national conscience. How fitting that the Sierra's most famous trail and one of its largest wilderness areas are both tributes to him.

By 1895, Solomons had discovered a route from Yosemite to the southern end of the San Joaquin drainage. Eight years after his inspiration to build the trail, Solomons had saved the money and procured the free time to begin scouting this route. During the summers of 1892, 1894, and 1895, he took extensive trips into the High Sierra and mapped a route from Yosemite Valley south to Evolution Basin. However, he was unable to find a stock-passable route across the Goddard Divide. Instead, he climbed through boulder fields and bushwhacked, without stock, through the Ionian Basin and down to the Middle Fork of the Kings River. Little Joe Le Conte accompanied him for part of the 1892 expedition, and in 1896, he followed a path similar to Solomons's from Yosemite to the Goddard Divide. There, he, too, failed to see today's Muir Pass as a navigable route and instead led his party far to the west and into the North Fork of the Kings River.

In contrast to the northern areas, the headwaters of the Kings River presented a barrier to crest-parallel travel for many years. It remained a challenge to find routes crossing the Kings-San Joaquin Divide, the Kings-Kern Divide, and the divides between the many forks of the Kings. Instead, parties accessed the region by traveling up the river drainages: The route from Cedar Grove to Bullfrog Lake and over Kearsarge Pass, and the route from Cedar Grove over Granite Pass and into the Middle Fork of the Kings River, were both stock-accessible and had already been traveled for many years by sheepherders.

It was by these routes that Bolton Brown entered the Sierra when he made long excursions into the South and Middle Forks of the Kings River (1895 and 1899) and the headwaters of the Kern (1896). Atypical for the period, he was often accompanied by his wife, Lucy, and, in 1899, also by their daughter, Eleanor. For JMT hikers, their most significant explorations included the discovery of Glen Pass (or Blue Flower Pass, as he named it) and the Rae Lakes region. However, he and Lucy were also the first people since the Brewer survey to cross the Kings-Kern Divide, and Brown extensively explored the headwaters of the South Fork Kings River and Woods Creek drainages, climbing peaks wherever he went.

It was Le Conte who finished piecing together most of a route through the headwaters of the King's forks. By 1900, Brown had left for the East Coast, and Solomons was working in Alaska. During the early 1900s, Le Conte made numerous trips to scout for possible passes across which trails could be built, focusing his efforts on the Middle and South Forks of the Kings.

In 1907, a US Geological Survey party had succeeded in crossing the Goddard Divide (a.k.a. the Kings-San Joaquin Divide) with stock, via the route that is now Muir Pass. A route across this divide had been the missing link in Le Conte's route, and with this information, in 1908, he set out to travel from Yosemite to Kings Canyon. Excepting a detour up Cataract Creek, when their horses could not navigate what would come to be known as the Golden Staircase, the Le Conte party's route was very similar to what would become the John Muir Trail between Yosemite Valley and Vidette Meadow. Thereafter, he descended Bubbs Creek to Cedar Grove.

As the headwaters of the Kern are less rugged, routes parallel to the Sierra Crest were easily found. Indeed, by 1908, the Kern River drainage was well-mapped, numerous parties had already climbed Mt. Whitney, and a rough use trail formed from Crabtree Meadow to Mt. Whitney's summit.

Ever more people entered the High Sierra with stock during the next years, often as part of the large Sierra Club summer excursions. But travel between the river basins was still difficult, and parties continued to enter from the west and visit single basins. In particular, Muir Pass, Mather Pass, and Forester Pass did not exist as navigable routes until the JMT was constructed, and most other passes sported only rough use trails.

In 1914, someone on an annual Sierra Club excursion suggested applying to the California legislature for funds to construct a high-mountain trail to facilitate access to the mountains. The following year, limited funds were procured in Sacramento. The legislature gave Wilbur McClure, the state engineer, the task of selecting a route from Yosemite Valley to Mt. Whitney. From Yosemite Valley to Vidette Meadow, the route he selected follows, with remarkable fidelity, the route identified by Solomons and Le Conte. To the south, he initially selected a route through Center Basin, over Junction Pass to the east side of the crest, and back across the drainage divide at Shepherd Pass, as no navigable routes were known across the precipitous Kings-Kern Divide. Only late in the construction of the trail was Forester Pass "discovered" and the decision made to reroute the trail along this more direct route.

Many of the explorers' tales are written as articles in old *Sierra Club Bulletins*, other magazines, or in published journals, gaining them fame for their efforts. Less flashy, less recorded, but equally important are the efforts of the many men who built the trail. By the end of your walk, you will appreciate the effort expended to dynamite cliffs and build switchbacks through the never-ending talus fields encountered over most passes.

Impressively, a rough trail in two sections, from Yosemite to Grouse Meadow (Middle Fork of Kings), and from Vidette Meadow (Bubbs Creek) to Mt. Whitney, was constructed within two years of funding. This included completely new stretches of trail over Muir Pass and Junction Pass. However, hikers had to detour to Simpson Meadow along the Middle Fork of the Kings and then across Granite Pass to Cedar Grove to bypass the Golden Staircase and Mather Pass. (Once good sections of trail existed over Pinchot Pass and Glen Pass, Cartridge Creek and Cartridge Pass were used to cross between the Middle and South Forks of the Kings.) Over the next many years, new stretches were built and rough sections were improved as funds became available. The trail to the summit of Mt. Whitney was completed in 1930, Forester Pass was finished in 1931 (only a year after the route was discovered), and the final section, the Golden Staircase, was completed in 1938.

Plants

Plant communities are generally defined by the species that dominates a particular community. At the most general level, the entire JMT is either beneath conifer cover or traversing terrain that does not support tree cover. Only on the first climb out of Yosemite Valley are deciduous trees a significant component. More specifically, the Sierra Nevada's forests can be divided into three zones: the mixed conifer zone, which extends to approximately 6500 feet; the upper montane zone, which extends from 6500 feet to 9000 or 10,000 feet; and the subalpine zone, which extends up to timberline. Above these is the alpine zone, where no trees grow. Only the first 5 miles of the JMT fall within the mixed conifer belt; the remainder of the trail is in the upper montane zone and above, and it is there we focus our attention.

The upper montane zone spans a wide range of elevations and which conifer species are dominant changes dramatically across this elevation gradient. At the lowest elevations, white fir is dominant, but with increasing elevation, red fir and western white pine become ever more common. At these same elevations, Jeffrey pines are present where the terrain is drier and rockier; usually, they stand alone or in small groups. As you move yet higher, western white pine and lodgepole pine intermingle, transitioning to nearly pure lodgepole pine stands at the upper end of this zone. As you travel even higher, you enter the subalpine zone. Whitebark pines dominate these highest

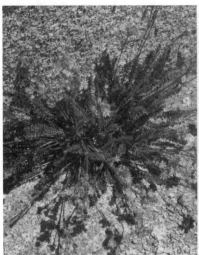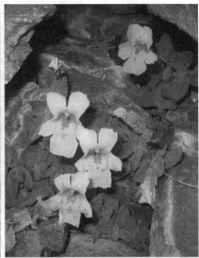

Club-moss ivesia (left) and mountain monkeyflower

elevation stands. In the alpine zone, the growing season is too short and the winter climate too extreme to support the growth of trees. Here you will see only small shrubs, herbs, and grasses, and the higher you climb, the smaller they will become.

In addition to elevation, slope aspect and latitude also affect which tree species will dominate. For instance, mountain hemlock is common in the north, often forming nearly mono-specific stands on north-facing slopes, but this species disappears as you move south. In contrast, fox-tail pine first appears south of Pinchot Pass and, under certain conditions, replaces the lodgepole forests by the time you reach Mt. Whitney. Some general characteristics to identify each of the conifer species are provided in the chart on page 33.

Of course, in addition to the conifer species, you will walk past at least 500 species of other trees, shrubs, herbs, and grasses on your journey. Most of these species are even pickier than the trees about the slope exposure, moisture availability, soil type, and more: Species may prefer wet meadows, dry meadows, seeps, stream banks, the edges of lakes, dry slopes, the base of boulders, cracks in boulders, talus piles, sandy flats, or some other specific habitat. And since most occur only at specific elevations, it is no wonder there are so many of them. Sporadically through the text, I describe some of the species you pass, a few at a time, allowing you to slowly build up your repertoire. Should you see all 120 of the species described in the text, you will have identified many of the Sierra Nevada's most common high-elevation species.

Common Conifers along the JMT

Note: Other than the first or last 6 miles of your hike, there are nine conifers that you will encounter frequently. They are each easily identified by the number of needles per group, cone size, and elevation range. Here, they are sorted by elevation range.

Common Name	Scientific Name	Needles		Cones		Elevation Range	Other
		Number	Length	Length	Shape		
White Fir	*Abies concolor*	1	1.25–2.25"	3–5"	Cylindrical, bulky	3000–8000'*	Cones never fall to ground intact.
Red Fir	*Abies magnificata*	1	0.6–1.25"	5–8"	Cylindrical, bulky	5000–9000'	Cones never fall to ground intact.
Jeffrey Pine	*Pinus jeffreyi*	3	8–10"	6–10"	Oval	6000–9000'	Cones' tips turned inward.
Western Juniper	*Juniperus occidentalis*	Tight scales		Small blue "berry"		7000–10,000'	Red, scaly bark.
Western White Pine	*Pinus monticola*	5	2–4"	4–8"	Cylindrical	7500–10,500'	Airy appearance.
Mountain Hemlock	*Tsuga mertensiana*	1	0.6–0.8"	1.6–3"	Oblong	8000–11,000'	More common in north.
Lodgepole Pine	*Pinus contorta*	2	1–3"	<2"	Round	6500–11,000'	Scaly bark, abundant cones.
Foxtail Pine	*Pinus balfouriana*	5	0.6–1.5"	2.5–7"	Cylindrical	9000–11,500'	Only south of Pinchot Pass.
Whitebark Pine	*Pinus albicaulis*	5	1.5–2.5"	2–3.5"	Slightly elongated	9500–12,000'	

* Occasionally higher

Animals

Birds, mammals, reptiles, amphibians, fish, and, of course, a great diversity of insects make their home in the High Sierra. Like the plants, animals are found in specific habitats.

Birds

Well over 100 species of birds have been spotted along the JMT. If you wish to end your hike with such an impressively long list, you are likely a birder, carrying binoculars, a bird book, and planning your layover days at the lowest-elevation habitats. Anyone else who keeps their eyes open can expect to see somewhere between 20 and 30 species along the way. In the text, I make note of 30 different bird species that are most common in the different habitats you pass through. At lower elevations, my descriptions include only the more common species, while the list is more exhaustive at the higher elevations; few species live above 10,000 feet and, as the tree cover thins, they become increasingly conspicuous.

Mammals

A large number of mammals live in the Sierra Nevada, but with the exception of many rodents, a few members of the rabbit family, deer, and bears, they do a good job of remaining hidden.

Among rodents, those you are mostly likely to see are the species active during the daytime: yellow-bellied marmots; chickarees, a small, dark-colored, and very loud tree squirrel; three species of ground squirrels, California (or Beechey), Belding's, and golden-mantled; and up to eight species of chipmunks. California ground squirrels, regularly occurring up 8000 feet and on occasion up to above 10,000 feet, are grayish-brown, with a light grey patch on the back of their necks, and a long, furry trail. In contrast, Belding's ground squirrels, occupying dry flats and meadows from 6000 to 11,500 feet, are a lighter, brown-beige color and have a short, nearly furless tail. Golden-mantled ground squirrels, which are found from 6000 feet to above timberline, look like overgrown chipmunks but lack the characteristic face stripes. Two members of the rabbit family that occur in the High Sierra are the pika, a little round critter with Mickey Mouse ears that lives in high-elevation talus piles, and the large, white-tailed jackrabbit.

As for large mammals, the mule deer is common throughout the Sierra Nevada, except over the highest passes. So-called timberline bucks venture up to and even above treeline. Black bears, despite their name, come in a great variety of colors. They range throughout the Sierra Nevada and, over the years, at increasingly high elevations. Luckily, you need only be concerned about your food, as this species is not aggressive toward humans. Nonetheless, should a bear get hold of your food, don't try to wrestle it away—that food now belongs to the bear. While many carnivore species inhabit the High Sierra, the only one you are likely to see is the coyote, active at dawn, dusk, and occasionally even midday. Their loud choruses can be both eerie and engaging.

Each year, a few lucky hikers, usually peak-baggers climbing talus slopes, get to see the Sierra Nevada bighorn sheep. The sheep in the Sierra Nevada are a distinct subspecies: They are genetically distinct from the bighorn sheep living just across the Owens Valley in the White Mountains.

Today, bighorn sheep live in only five regions of the Sierra Nevada—a fraction of the territory they inhabited when Europeans first visited. The Europeans brought along domestic sheep—and their diseases, which were rapidly transmitted to the native sheep, decimating their populations. By the early 1970s, only two groups remained, one whose range stretched between Taboose and Kearsarge passes, and one that lived on and around Mt. Williamson, near Shepherd Pass. Thanks to reintroduction efforts, there are now also populations of sheep on the peaks east of Tuolumne Meadows (the Mono Basin unit), on the Wheeler Crest, a region well east of Mono Creek and Bear Creek; and on Mt. Langley, south of Mt. Whitney. In the early 1990s, sheep in all

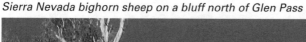

Sierra Nevada bighorn sheep on a bluff north of Glen Pass

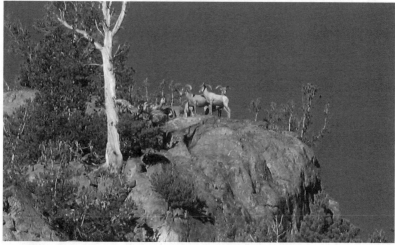

five regions experienced severe population declines, reaching a population low in 1995. Since then, their population has been rebounding, and we can hope that their numbers continue to increase in the coming years. After all, as John Muir wrote, they are the "bravest of all the Sierra mountaineers," and they exist only in these mountains.

Along the JMT, you are most likely to see sheep in the vicinity of Pinchot Pass and down toward the White Fork crossing, as you hike through Rae Lakes and over Glen Pass, and possibly south of Forester Pass. But don't set your heart on finding sheep: In more than 600 days of hiking in the Sierra Nevada, including ascents of nearly every peak in sheep country, I have seen groups only twice. Yes, *twice!* The rest of the time, I found their little piles of, often fresh, droppings deposited on talus sloes, taunting me to stare ever harder at the landscape. All I can do is pass on the advice of the researchers: Hunt for the granite boulders with legs.

A few more words regarding sheep biology: The sheep require open, steep, rocky habitat. The cliff bands provide protection from predators and, amazingly, on the adjacent talus slopes grow sufficient plants to provide their nutrition. Their favorite foods include those plants you will see only over the highest passes: alpine gold, sky pilot, and mountain sorrel.

During summer, the males and females live in separate herds. The females and their lambs tend to live on the higher, safer slopes, while the males are more likely to descend toward lake basins to feed. It is therefore the males you are more likely to see as you cross passes along the JMT.

Reptiles, Amphibians, and Fish

Not many reptiles and amphibians inhabit the high elevations of the Sierra Nevada, but you may encounter a few along the JMT. Western terrestrial garter snakes can occur in wet areas up to at least 10,000 feet, and western rattlesnakes can occur as high as 8000 feet, but they are much more common at lower elevations. As for amphibians, the Mt. Lyell salamander inhabits seeps up to at least 12,000 feet, but it is rarely seen. Four species of frogs also live in the High Sierra, and the range for each extends toward the 12,000-foot mark: the Pacific tree frog, the Yosemite toad, the western toad, and the mountain yellow-legged frog. Of these, the Pacific tree frog is the most common. This species is just larger that your thumbnail and sports a characteristic black eye stripe. Its tadpoles are commonly seen in warm, shallow, temporary bodies of water.

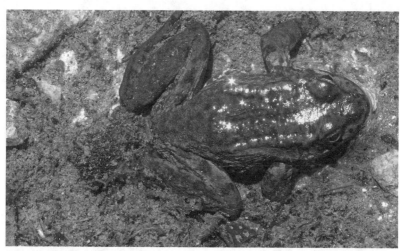

Mountain yellow-legged frog

The mountain yellow-legged frog is the Sierra Nevada amphibian that has garnered the greatest attention in the last decades. This large frog, with a mottled brown coloration pattern and light undersides, breeds only in high-elevation lakes. These are the same lakes into which non-native trout species have been transplanted, and the tadpoles make a tasty and captive treat for those fish. Unlike the other frog species, the mountain yellow-legged tadpoles take approximately four years to metamorphose into adult frogs and therefore must live in the larger, deeper lakes that do not freeze solid in winter. In order to increase frog habitat, the national parks, and increasingly the national forests, have stopped stocking fish in wilderness lakes and have even removed fish from a subset of lakes. Unfortunately, in recent years, a fungal parasite, a type of chytrid, is threatening to decimate nearly all populations along the length of the Sierra Nevada. You may be lucky and pass one of the lakes along the JMT whose shallow shorelines are still teeming with the 2- to 4–inch-long tadpoles (many different sizes and stages of development can be seen simultaneously). And please note that amphibians absorb chemicals through their skins, so if you see amphibians in a body of water, be extra careful not to contaminate it with sunscreen, insect repellant, soap, etc. More information is available at: www.yosemite.org/naturenotes/SteckelChytrid1.htm.

The five species of trout that inhabit the waters along the JMT have been introduced along almost the entire length of the JMT. The only exception is the presence of rainbow trout in the Merced River downstream of Vernal Fall—less than a mile of your total journey. The steep waterfalls and cascades along the western and eastern slopes of the Sierra Nevada prevented fish from establishing themselves at higher elevations. Stocking, beginning in the 1870s to create a food source in the otherwise "barren" Sierra Nevada lakes, rapidly changed this. As a result, rainbow trout (native to lower-elevation western Sierra Nevada rivers), golden trout (native to the southern Sierra Nevada), Lahontan cutthroat trout (native to some eastern Sierra Nevada drainages), brown trout (native to Europe), and brook trout (native to the eastern US) are now common throughout the Sierra Nevada's waters. Although non-native, these fish are tasty, and with a fishing rod and a fishing permit, you can easily supplement your daily dinners.

Geology

At first pass, the Sierra Nevada is a long spine of granite, formed deep in the Earth when the Farallon Plate collided into the North American Plate 120 million to 80 million years ago. But upon closer inspection, variation in rock types are evident.

First, the appearance of the granite changes between locations. The chemical composition of granite is readily discernable by determining the relative abundance of its five main minerals—quartz, two types of feldspar (potassium-feldspar, and a more sodium/calcium-rich feldspar called plagioclase), biotite, and hornblende. Quartz and plagioclase are white in color, potassium-feldspar is a light pink, and biotite and hornblende are black. Which minerals form is in turn determined by the chemical composition of the magma that cooled to form the granite, and you will indeed pass granite boulders whose color varies from quite white to containing a large percent of dark minerals.

Second, along the JMT, you will pass long stretches of non-granitic rock. Volcanic deposits in the vicinity of the Mammoth Crest and Devils Postpile National Monument are less than 3 million years old. There are also several large regions of metamorphic rocks, including the Ritter Range, the Goddard Terrane (extending from Goddard Canyon up to the Mt. Goddard vicinity and south along the Black Divide), and the High Sierra Terrane (extending along the Sierra Crest from near Mather Pass south to Glen Pass). The metamorphosed rock—sedimentary or volcanic rock that was subjected to high pressures or temperatures and hence recrystalized—is older than the granite. The volcanic precursors to the Goddard Terrane and the sedimentary precursors to the High Sierra Terrane both formed at their current locations and were metamorphosed during the creation and subsequent uplift of the granitic rocks.

Superimposed on the present rock are the geomorphic landforms, many glacial in origin. These are described in the text, as indicated in the chart below.

Index of Geological Features Described in Text

Glacial Features

Glacial Erratics – 76, 99, 106, 182, 188, 207
Glacial Polish – 106, 182
Hanging Valley – 105, 183
Little Ice Age – 75, 158
Moraine – 120, 132, 152, 166–167
Roche Moutonneé – 71, 213
Rock Glacier – 90, 125, 138, 158, 161, 195
Sierra Glaciation – 28, 67, 75, 106–107, 158, 182, 183, 208, 214
Unglaciated Topography – 106, 130, 154, 182

Non-Glacial Geomorphic Features

Avalanche Chutes – 106, 130, 149, 153, 154–160, 183
Domes – 64, 65, 71, 213, 218–219
Exfoliation – 65, 218–219
Fault Line, Kern – 129, 155
Joints – 67, 106, 130, 149, 214
Oxbow Lakes – 110, 177

Volcanic Features

Columnar Basalt – 84, 201
Devils Postpile – 84, 201
Lave Tubes – 85, 198
Mammoth Mountain – 86, 199–200
Pumice – 86, 197
Volcanic Activity – 78, 86, 199–200, 203

Metamorphic and Metavolcanic Rocks

Fracture Patterns – 103, 184
Goddard Terrane/ Ionian Basin – 107, 110, 115, 178, 184
High Sierra Terrane – 115, 171
Metamorphic Rock Decomposition – 117, 169
Ritter Range – 78, 86, 200, 203
Roof Pendants – 115, 171, 175
Tectonic Activity – 86, 107, 115, 171, 178, 200

Minerals

Epidote – 133, 151
Feldspar, Zoned – 135, 149
Potassium-Feldspar – 133, 151
Mineral Composition – 77, 99, 133, 151, 188, 207

CUMULATIVE
MILEAGE TABLE

Location	From North	Distance Between Points	From South
Happy Isles	0		218.5
		0.8	
Base of Vernal Fall	0.8		217.7
		0.2	
Mist Trail junction	1.0		217.5
		1.0	
Clark Point junction	2.0		216.5
		0.8	
Panorama Trail junction	2.8		215.7
		0.5	
Nevada Fall junction	3.3		215.2
		0.6	
Western Little Yosemite Valley junction	3.9		214.6
		0.6	
Northeastern Little Yosemite Valley junction	4.5		214.0
		1.5	
Half Dome junction	6.0		212.5
		0.5	
Clouds Rest junction	6.5		212.0
		1.9	
Merced Lake junction	8.4		210.1
		0.1	
Forsyth Trail junction	8.5		210.0
		4.6	
Sunrise Lakes junction	13.1		205.4
		0.9	
Echo Creek junction	14.0		204.5
		2.7	
Cathedral Pass	16.7		201.8
		1.1	
Lower Cathedral Lake junction	17.8		200.7
		0.5	
Mariposa-Tuolumne County Line	18.3		200.2
		2.4	
Cathedral Lakes Parking Area junction	20.7		197.8
		0.9	

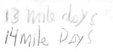

13 mile days
14 mile Days

Location	From North	Distance Between Points	From South
Western merge with alternate route	21.6		196.9
		0.6	
Parsons Lodge junction	22.2		196.3
		0.7	
Lembert Dome parking area	22.9		195.6
		1.1	
Tuolumne High Sierra Camp junction	24.0		194.5
		0.6	
Eastern merge with alternate route	24.6		193.9
		0.7	
Rafferty Creek junction	25.3		193.2
		4.2	
Evelyn Lake junction	29.5		189.0
		3.0	
Start of climb from Lyell Canyon (Lyell Forks)	32.5		186.0
		1.1	
Bridge across Lyell Forks of the Tuolumne	33.6		184.9
		1.0	
Wade across the Lyell Forks of the Tuolumne	34.6		183.9
		1.8	
Donohue Pass	36.4		182.1
		2.7	
Marie Lakes junction	39.1		179.4
		0.9	
Rush Creek junction	40.0		178.5
		0.3	
Davis Lakes junction	40.3		178.2
		1.0	
Island Pass	41.3		177.2
		1.8	
Thousand Island Lake junction	43.1		175.4
		2.2	
Garnet Lake junction	45.3		173.2
		2.4	
Lake Ediza junction	47.7		170.8
		0.9	
Shadow Lake junction	48.6		169.9
		1.5	
Rosalie Lake outlet	50.1		168.4
		0.6	
Gladys Lake	50.7		167.8
		2.3	
Trinity Lakes outlet crossing	53.0		165.5
		2.0	
Johnston Meadow	55.0		163.5
		0.6	
Beck Lakes junction	55.6		162.9
		0.7	
Northern Devils Postpile junction	56.3		162.2
		0.7	
Southern Devils Postpile junction	57.0		161.5
		1.2	
Rainbow Falls junction	58.2		160.3
		0.5	

Location	From North	Distance Between Points	From South
Reds Meadow junction	58.7		159.8
		3.1	
Crater Creek crossing at Red Cones	61.8		156.7
		0.9	
Mammoth Pass junction in Upper Crater Meadow	62.7		155.8
		1.1	
Madera-Fresno County Line	63.8		154.7
		0.9	
Deer Creek crossing	64.7		153.8
		5.6	
Duck Pass junction	70.3		148.2
		2.3	
Purple Lake outlet	72.6		145.9
		2.0	
Lake Virginia inlet	74.6		143.9
		2.0	
Tully Hole junction	76.6		141.9
		1.0	
Cascade Creek junction	77.6		140.9
		2.0	
Squaw Lake outlet	79.6		138.9
		0.5	
Goodale Pass junction	80.1		138.4
		1.0	
Silver Pass	81.1		137.4
		3.7	
Mott Lake junction	84.8		133.7
		1.4	
Mono Creek junction	86.2		132.3
		1.4	
Lake Edison junction	87.6		130.9
		4.6	
Bear Ridge junction	92.2		126.3
		2.1	
Bear Creek junction	94.3		124.2
		2.0	
Hilgard Fork junction	96.3		122.2
		1.2	
Bear Lakes junction	97.5		121.0
		1.1	
Three Island Lake junction	98.6		119.9
		0.3	
Rose Lake junction	98.9		119.6
		1.6	
Marie Lake outlet	100.5		118.0
		0.9	
Selden Pass	101.4		117.1
		3.6	
Senger Creek crossing	105.0		113.5
		2.1	
JMT northern cutoff	107.1		111.4
		1.7	
JMT southern cutoff	108.8		109.7
		1.8	

Location	From North	Distance Between Points	From South
Piute Creek junction	110.6		107.9
		3.5	
Goddard Creek junction	114.1		104.4
		1.5	
Wade across Evolution Creek	115.6		102.9
		2.4	
McClure Meadow ranger station	118.0		100.5
		5.2	
Evolution Lake inlet	123.2		95.3
		2.5	
Wanda Lake outlet	125.7		92.8
		2.2	
Muir Pass	127.9		90.6
		1.3	
Helen Lake outlet	129.2		89.3
		2.3	
Starrs Camp	131.5		87.0
		2.3	
Big Pete Meadow creek crossing	133.8		84.7
		1.9	
Bishop Pass junction	135.7		82.8
		3.4	
Middle Fork junction	139.1		79.4
		3.4	
Deer Meadow creek crossing	142.5		76.0
		3.5	
Lower Palisade Lake outlet	146.0		72.5
		3.6	
Mather Pass	149.6		68.9
		3.0	
South Fork Kings crossing at base of Upper Basin	152.6		65.9
		2.2	
Main South Fork Kings crossing	154.8		63.7
		1.5	
Taboose Pass junction	156.3		62.2
		1.0	
Crossing below Lake Marjorie	157.3		61.2
		2.1	
Pinchot Pass	159.4		59.1
		3.7	
Sawmill Pass junction	163.1		55.4
		3.5	
Woods Creek junction	166.6		51.9
		3.7	
Baxter Pass junction	170.3		48.2
		2.1	
Rae Lakes ranger station	172.4		46.1
		1.0	
60 Lakes Basin junction	173.4		45.1
		1.9	
Glen Pass	175.3		43.2
		2.0	
Kearsarge Pass junction	177.3		41.2
		0.3	

Location	From North	Distance Between Points	From South
Charlotte Lake junction	177.6		40.9
		0.5	
Bullfrog Lake junction	178.1		40.4
		1.3	
Bubbs Creek junction	179.4		39.1
		1.2	
Upper Vidette Meadow bear box	180.6		37.9
		2.1	
Center Basin Creek crossing	182.7		35.8
		3.1	
Lake at 12,250 feet	185.8		32.7
		1.3	
Forester Pass	187.1		31.4
		0.8	
Highest Tyndall Creek crossing	187.9		30.6
		3.6	
Lake South America junction	191.5		27.0
		0.3	
Shepherd Pass junction	191.8		26.7
		2.0	
Bighorn Plateau	193.8		24.7
		1.9	
Wright Creek crossing	195.7		22.8
		0.7	
High Sierra Trail junction	196.4		22.1
		1.5	
Ridge west of Mt. Young	197.9		20.6
		2.0	
PCT junction west of Crabtree Meadows	199.9		18.6
		0.8	
Crabtree Meadow and ranger station	200.7		17.8
		1.4	
Timberline Lake outlet	202.1		16.4
		1.3	
Arctic Lake outlet creek	203.4		15.1
		2.9	
Mt. Whitney Trail junction	206.3		12.2
		1.9	
Mt. Whitney	208.2		10.3
		2.1	
Trail Crest	210.3		8.2
		2.3	
Trail Camp	212.6		5.9
		1.9	
Mirror Lake	214.5		4.0
		0.4	
Outpost Camp	214.9		3.6
		1.1	
Lone Pine Lake junction	216.0		2.5
		1.6	
North Fork Lone Pine Creek crossing	217.6		0.9
		0.9	
Whitney Portal	218.5		0.0

MAPS

About Map Sections

The following topographic maps are from the John Muir Trail Map-Pack by Tom Harrison Maps. While these maps are divided into 13 sections, please note that they are not divided in the same way as the 13 sections described in the book. The 13 trail sections in the book correspond with 13 major drainages that the JMT passes through.

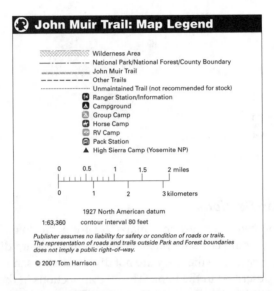

John Muir Trail: Map Legend

Wilderness Area
National Park/National Forest/County Boundary
John Muir Trail
Other Trails
Unmaintained Trail (not recommended for stock)
Ranger Station/Information
Campground
Group Camp
Horse Camp
RV Camp
Pack Station
High Sierra Camp (Yosemite NP)

0   0.5   1   1.5   2 miles

0   1   2   3 kilometers

1927 North American datum

1:63,360   contour interval 80 feet

Publisher assumes no liability for safety or condition of roads or trails.
The representation of roads and trails outside Park and Forest boundaries
does not imply a public right–of–way.

© 2007 Tom Harrison

John Muir Trail: Index to Map Panels and Trailheads

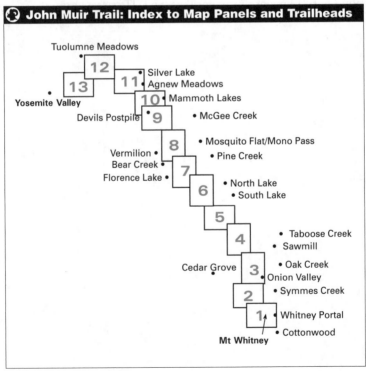

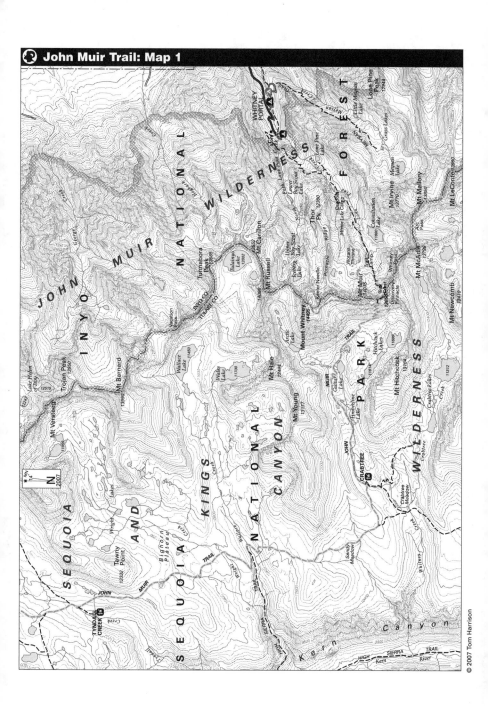

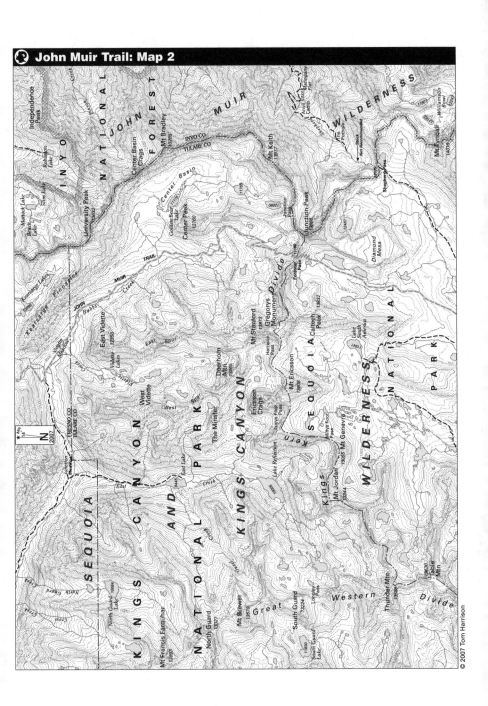

John Muir Trail: Map 2

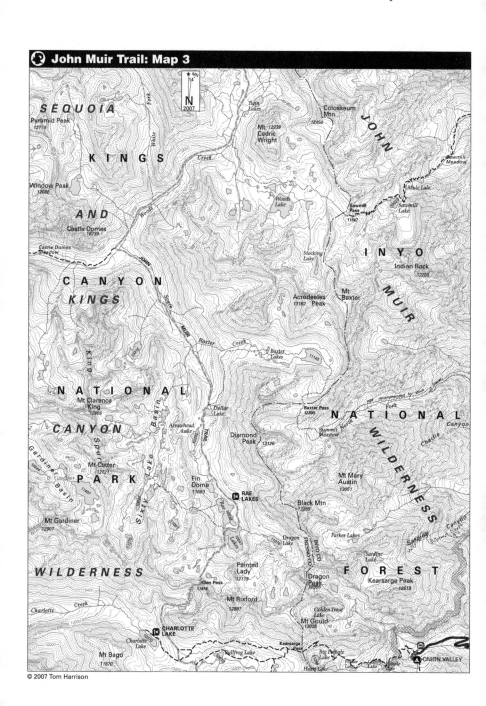

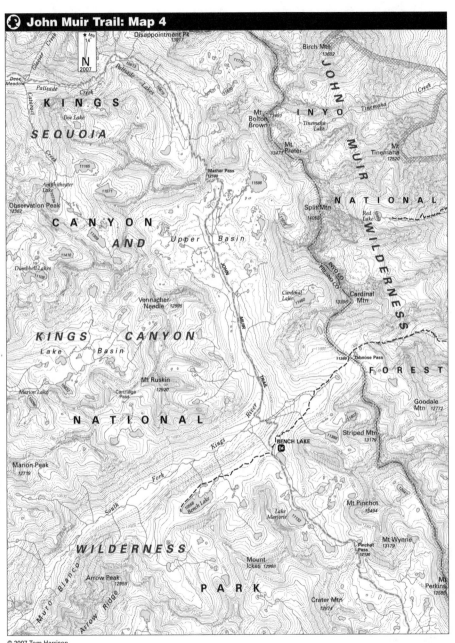

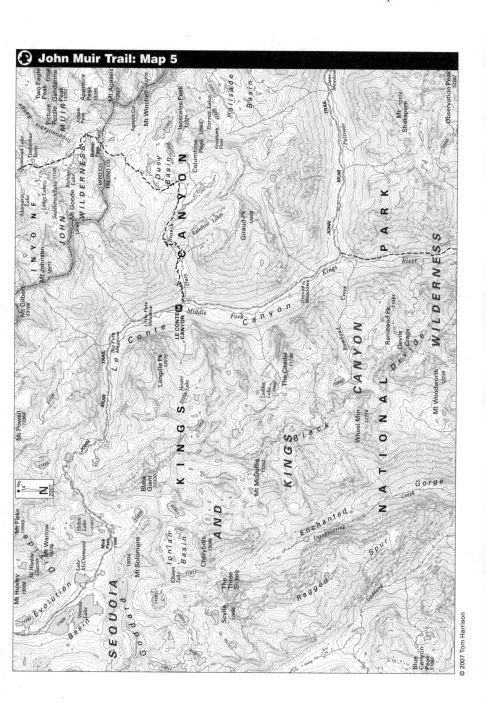

John Muir Trail: Map 5

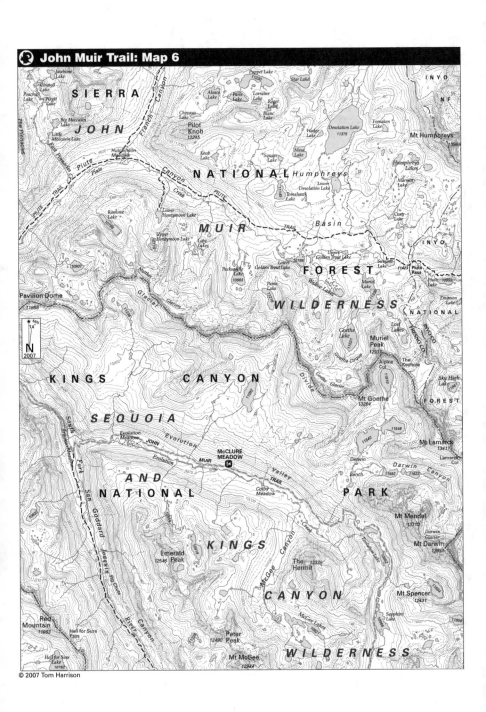

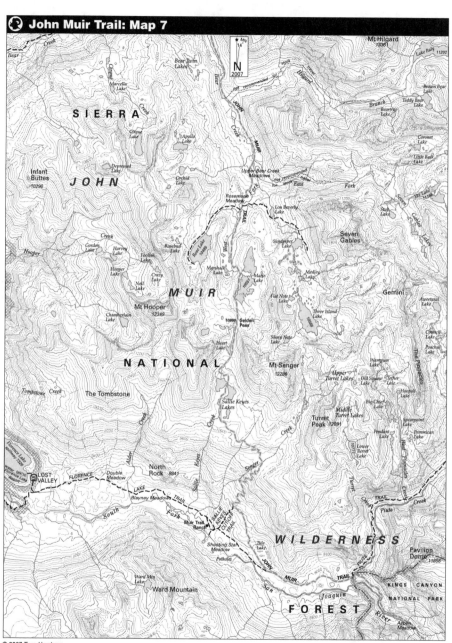

John Muir Trail: Map 7

© 2007 Tom Harrison

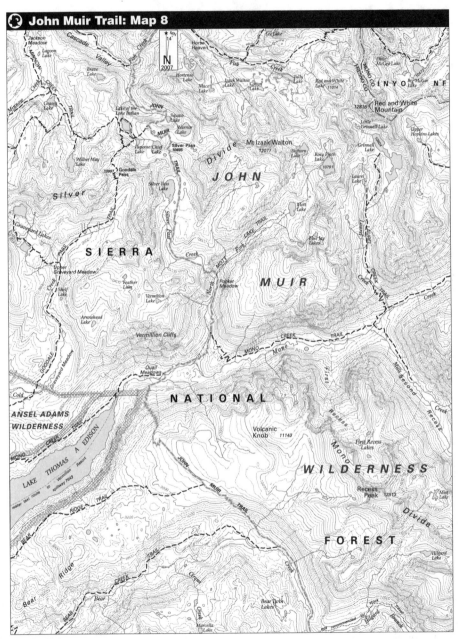

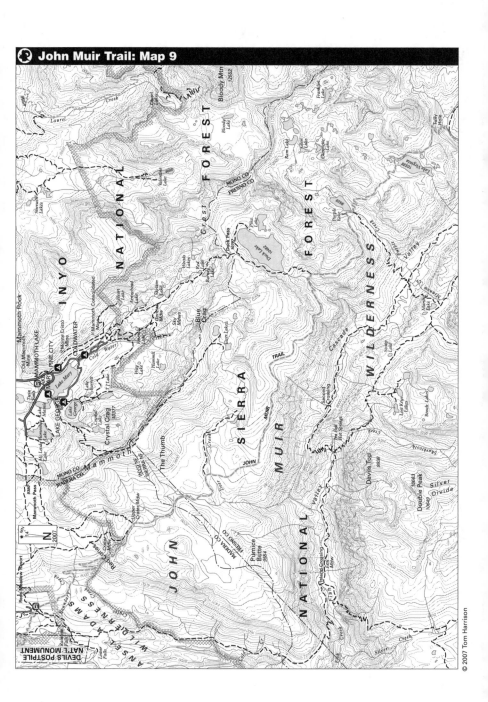

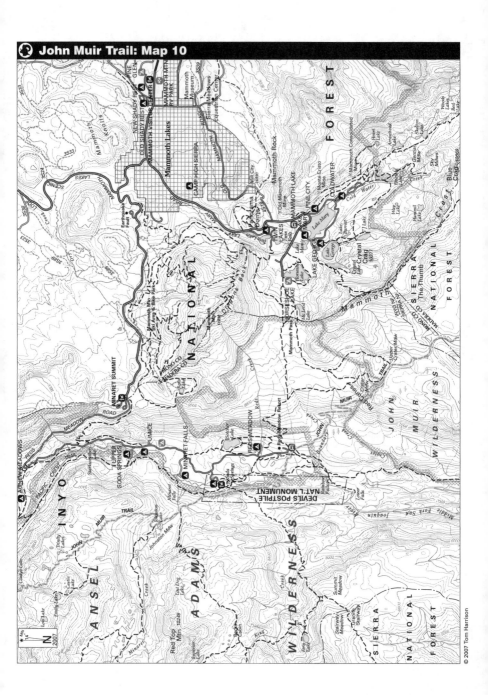

John Muir Trail: Map 10

© 2007 Tom Harrison

John Muir Trail: Map 11

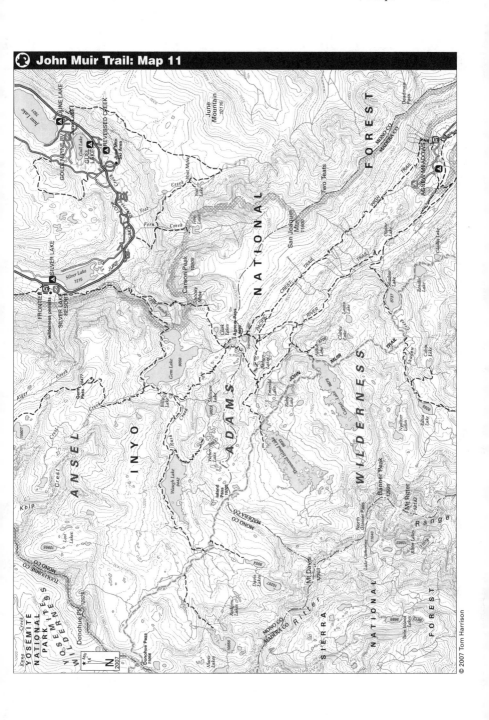

© 2007 Tom Harrison

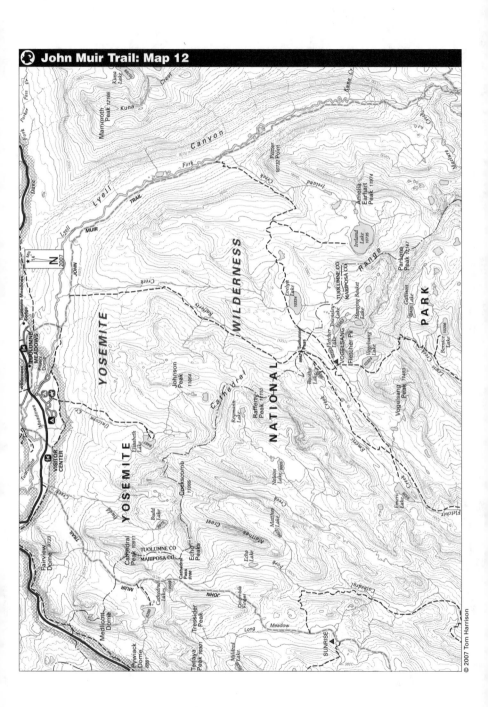

John Muir Trail: Map 12

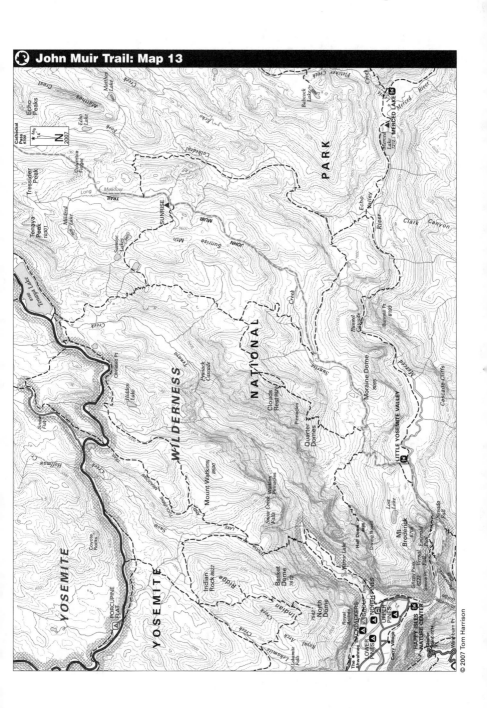

John Muir Trail: Map 13

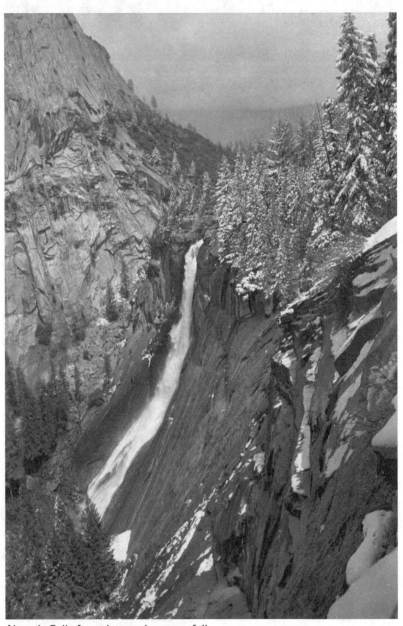

Nevada Fall after a late spring snowfall

NORTH TO SOUTH:

YOSEMITE VALLEY TO WHITNEY PORTAL

SECTION 1.

Happy Isles to Tuolumne–Mariposa County Line—Merced River

At its start, the asphalt-surfaced trail climbs steeply southward and upward on the east wall of the river canyon. You'll have plenty of company from here to the junction with the trail to Half Dome. The route curves around the base of Sierra Point, a popular vista point until a rockfall closed the trail many years ago. Continue eastward, high above the turbulent Merced River. You descend briefly to cross the river on a stout footbridge [4390′ – 0.8/0.8] offering a superb view of Vernal Fall; be sure to pull out your camera. Across the bridge are restrooms and a drinking fountain that has been refurbished with spouts for both drinking and filling water bottles. This is the last treated water

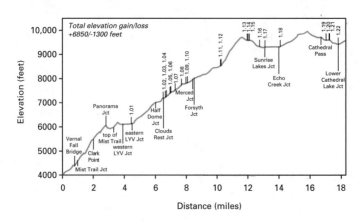

until Tuolumne Meadows. A short distance above the bridge is a junction, where the Mist Trail continues straight ahead and the JMT turns south to begin switchbacking up the canyon's steep south wall [4600′ – 0.2/1.0]. The Mist Trail skirts the edge of the river, following stairs up the steep river channel to the top of Vernal Fall. This scenic route is considerably shorter and steeper, and in early and midseason, it is so wet from spray that you will reach the top drenched. Nonetheless, if you are up for the challenge of hauling your pack up this route, it is well worth the views—and the hot sun will quickly dry your clothes. From the top

Location	Elevation	Distance from Previous Point	Cumulative Distance	UTM Coordinates
Happy Isles	4035	—	0	11S 274640E 4178853N
Base of Vernal Fall	4390	0.8	0.8	11S 275238E 4178312N
Mist Trail junction	4600	0.2	1.0	11S 275458E 4178298N
Clark Point junction	5480	1.0	2.0	11S 275787E 4178164N
Panorama Trail junction	6040	0.8	2.8	11S 276617E 4177802N
Nevada Fall junction	5980	0.5	3.3	11S 277073E 4178263N
Western Little Yosemite Valley junction	6100	0.6	3.9	11S 277749E 4178733N
Northeastern Little Yosemite Valley junction	6140	0.6	4.5	11S 278453E 4179139N
Half Dome junction	7015	1.5	6.0	11S 278771E 4180309N
Clouds Rest junction	7190	0.5	6.5	11S 279498E 4180201N
Merced Lake junction	7960	1.9	8.4	11S 281692E 4181495N
Forsyth Trail junction	8010	0.1	8.5	11S 281726E 4181593N
Sunrise Lakes junction	9320	4.6	13.1	11S 285841E 4185488N
Echo Creek junction	9320	0.9	14.0	11S 286133E 4186544N
Cathedral Pass	9700	2.7	16.7	11S 287535E 4190040N
Lower Cathedral Lake junction	9425	1.1	17.8	11S 287610E 4191528N
Mariposa-Tuolumne County Line	9570	0.5	18.3	11S 287795E 4192140N

SEE MAP 13

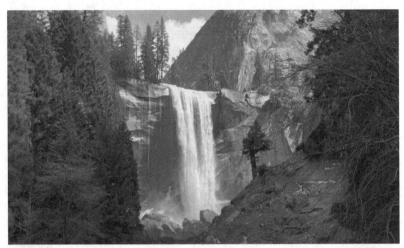

Vernal Fall

of Vernal Fall, you could choose to climb up to Clark Point to rejoin the JMT sooner, or continue ascending the Mist Trail to the top of Nevada Fall. The two trails rejoin at the top of Nevada Fall.

Assuming you continue up the JMT, you will shortly pass a signed horse trail coming in from the west, and begin ascending switchbacks. The tree species on this slope are unique to this stretch of the JMT and disappear as you climb higher. Douglas fir is the main conifer species, while three broadleaf species are California black oak, identified by their large, lobed leaves; big-leaf maples; and California bay-laurels, which have long, skinny, leathery, and highly aromatic leaves. Meanwhile, the ever-squawking Steller's jays, dark blue birds with a black crest, will follow you several thousand feet higher. You will undoubtedly stop and watch these, as the switchbacks seem interminable and are tough on your feet, since many were once paved. After the climb, you will enjoy a break at the Clark Point junction to take in the view of the waterfalls and the surrounding canyon [5480' – 1.0/2.0]. Continue upward on the JMT, first on switchbacks and then along a walled-in section of trail that clings to the cliff. In late season, damp sections of this trail are colored by California fuchsias, a low-growing shrub with bright red, tubular flowers, and grass-of-Parnassus, creamy white, five-petal flowers on tall stems. The view from the west end of the walled traverse is spectacular. In the distance is the rounded backside of Half Dome, and to the east, Nevada Fall drops 594 feet. Mt. Broderick and Liberty Cap are the two prominent domes across the drainage. While these domes were glaciated, their rounded tops actually exist due to

SEE MAP 13

exfoliation of their constituent granite; imagine the peeling-off layers of an onion. Shortly after the traverse, you pass a signed junction with the Panorama Trail [6040′ – 0.8/2.8].

The trail bends to the northeast, leading to the top of Nevada Fall. A sturdy footbridge leads over the raging waters, after which the trail passes a spur to a fenced vista point, follows a line of rocks across slabs, and zigzags down to meet the upper end of the Mist Trail near some restrooms [5980′ – 0.5/3.3]. You now climb a short distance up sandy, rocky switchbacks, on which vegetation includes canyon live oak; Fremont silktassel, with long, dangling tassels of flowers; black oak; and, occasionally, a towering Jeffrey pine, with long needles and large cones. After a short climb, you drop into Little Yosemite Valley, your first flat section of trail, and traipse along the riverbank. In early season, the western azaleas that line the river are thickly covered in aromatic white flowers. At a junction [6100′ – 0.6/3.9], the JMT takes the right fork, while the left fork is a shortcut, and the two merge again a little north of the Little Yosemite Valley camping area. The JMT, mostly under dense forest, roughly parallels the now unseen river, which it is separated from by a crude log fence. In early season, you may see the peculiar red snowplant that is non-photosynthetic but obtains nutrients from nearby tree roots. Soon, the JMT turns north (left) at a junction and passes by the large Little Yosemite Valley camping area, the first legal camping since Yosemite Valley. Here there are toilets and bear boxes. Soon after the toilets, you re-intersect the shortcut trail [6140′ – 0.6/4.5] and resume climbing.

In stretches, you climb at a steady grade through a predominately white fir forest, but elsewhere are flat stretches lined with magnificent incense cedars with shaggy red bark and minute scaly leaves. A few sugar pines, with enormous, elongated cones, and Jeffrey pines also grace the forest. The diminutive pygmy nuthatch, with a straight, chisel-like bill, and the curved-billed brown creeper live in these forests, the former circling down, and the latter circling up tree trunks in search of insects. This is also home to the blue grouse, which is often perched high in the trees. In early summer, the *whoop-whoop-whoop* of the males, followed by a sudden flurry of wing beats, is likely to startle you. The JMT next meets the lateral to Half Dome [7015′ – 1.5/6.0], an incredible 4-mile round trip that shouldn't be missed (see Appendix E). The JMT turns east and traverses to Sunrise Creek on a dry slope with dense scrub cover: The underlying slabs are close to the surface, and in many places there is insufficient soil depth for trees. In half a mile, the JMT meets the trail to Clouds Rest [7190′ – 0.5/6.5], another worthwhile detour with outstanding views of Yosemite Valley, Half Dome, and the Yosemite high country (see Appendix E).

There are a few campsites near the junction, a large camping area just a bit farther along the JMT in a flat forest opening along the banks of Sunrise Creek, and an improved site on the low ridge to the northeast of Sunrise Creek. The JMT now follows Sunrise Creek, passing occasional campsites between the trail and the stream. Just before you cross Sunrise Creek, a collection of use trails leads north to campsites atop a small knob that have delightful views toward Half Dome and Mt. Starr King, a dome south of the Merced River canyon. The trail continues to climb through white fir forest, with openings sporting Jeffrey pines. Creeping snowberry, with small, pink, tubular flowers and slightly lobed leaves, is a common ground cover throughout these dry forests. As you ascend, the white fir are slowly replaced by red fir, with much shorter needles and often redder bark. The cones of this species differ as well, but these are always consumed by critters before dropping from the trees, and therefore are of little use to hikers for identification. A few more campsites appear after you diverge from the main Sunrise Creek and intersect a small tributary. You cross the creek and shortly reach the junction first with a trail to Merced Lake [7960' – 1.9/8.4] and immediately thereafter with the Forsyth Trail [8010' – 0.1/8.5].

For the next mile, the trail diverges from Sunrise Creek, crossing over open flats before reentering dry, bare, red fir forest. Where the trail bends north, a few campsites emerge: the first along the banks of a potentially dry tributary and others where you again cross Sunrise Creek. These are your last campsites for several miles, as you now begin the climb up Sunrise Mountain. Red fir, western white pine, western juniper, and Jeffrey pines are all present along the ensuing climb. Western white pine has mid-sized needles in groups of five, arranged on the branch in a way that gives them an airy appearance. Higher still, you enter the first lodgepole pine forest along the JMT. This species will dominate along much of the trail. Lodgepole pines are characterized by small, round cones that are always abundant around tree trunks, needles in clusters of two, and fine-scaly bark. Shortly, you cross a shallow, sandy ridge and descend to a meadow, alongside which there are several campsites. A common shrub throughout this area is alpine prickly currant, with prickly trailing stems, slightly lobed leaves, and edible red berries. Along the entire length of the JMT, this species is abundant from the montane to the alpine regions, often forming thickets along the ground in lodgepole forests. The trail crosses another sandy ridge and descends toward Sunrise High Sierra Camp.

SEE MAP 13

En route, you cross one small tributary where there is a small campsite among mountain hemlock trees. These short-needled conifers with small, elongate cones prefer cooler, north-facing slopes and gradually diminish in abundance to the south. But I leave it to John Muir to further describe his favorite tree: "The hemlock spruce is the most singularly beautiful of all the California coniferæ. So slender is its axis at the top, that it bends over and droops like the stalk of a nodding lily. The branches droop also, and divide into innumerable slender, waving sprays, which are arranged in a varied, eloquent harmony that is wholly indescribable." Be sure to spend one night on your walk beneath their elegant boughs!

A short descent brings you to L-shaped Long Meadow and the junction with the trail to Sunrise Lakes and Clouds Rest [9320' – 4.6/13.1]. Many campsites, bear boxes, and a pit toilet can be found a short distance up this trail. A spur trail to Sunrise High Sierra Camp lays a short stretch ahead; the camp has supplies only for its guests, who put their names into the reservation lottery months in advance. Be sure to enjoy the spectacular views south to the Clark Range and southeast to Mt. Florence before turning north up Long Meadow, which you skirt on sandy flats along its western edge. Near the Echo Creek Trail junction [9320' – 0.9/14.0], you briefly enter forest and pass a small campsite to the west of the trail, before re-emerging into ever-continuing Long Meadow. You now see notably steep Columbia Finger straight ahead. This spire of jointed rock once arose above the surrounding ice fields. Summiting Columbia Finger requires a bit of scrambling, but sports an excellent view if you have time for a detour (see Appendix E).

Beyond Long Meadow, you continue the climb toward Cathedral Pass, through open, sandy lodgepole forest. Alongside boulders, you will find mountain pride penstemon, one of the most common species both here and in the subalpine region. It is easily identified by vast blooms of tubular, bright magenta flowers decorating a low-growing shrub with slightly serrate leaves. When you reach a sandy saddle, stop and enjoy the view of the Cathedral Range: the milelong, knife-edge Matthes Crest to your east, the Echo Peaks and Cathedral Peak to the northeast, and Columbia Finger and Tresidder Peak to the west. For each peak, note that the lower reaches are smooth and steep, having been rolled over by glaciers, while the summits are jagged spires of jointed rock. You now descend the eastern shoulder of Tresidder Peak toward the broad saddle called Cathedral Pass [9700' – 2.7/16.7] and into the shallow cirque cradling the upper Cathedral Lake. The lake is nestled in a large meadow and surrounded by the steep lower walls

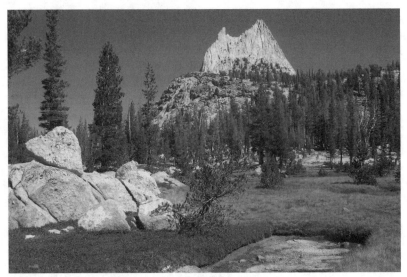

Cathedral Peak viewed from the upper Cathedral Lake

of Tresidder Peak and the Echo Peaks. A handful of campsites can be found to the east of the trail and in trees at the northern end of the lake. Campfires are prohibited both here and at the lower Cathedral Lake. You continue descending through mixed lodgepole and hemlock forest. The low-growing dwarf bilberry, a type of blueberry with small, ovate leaves and bell-shaped flowers, dominates the edge of meadows and wet sections of forest floor, but unfortunately, it rarely bares fruit. Shortly, you reach a lateral trail to the lower Cathedral Lake [9425' – 1.1/17.8], where you will find additional campsites, your last before Tuolumne Meadows. You now make a gradual climb through open lodgepole forest and then onto a sandy shoulder, the whole while traversing below Cathedral Peak. In 1869, John Muir was the first to climb this magnificent peak, via the slabs on the west face, the route at which you are gazing. Shortly, you reach a seemingly un-noteworthy saddle, but this pass is the divide between the Merced and Tuolumne river drainages [9570' – 0.5/18.3]. There is no marker indicating when you cross the drainage divide and it is difficult to decide when the grade becomes "downhill," but the results farther downstream couldn't be more dramatic: Water flowing into the Cathedral Lakes drains into Tenaya Lake and then down Tenaya Canyon to Yosemite Valley, while water to the north flows down the Tuolumne River to Hetch Hetchy Reservoir and the plumbing of San Francisco.

SEE MAP 12

SECTION 2.

Tuolumne-Mariposa County Line to Donohue Pass—Tuolumne River

Slowly, the slope increases, dropping more steeply past a robust spring and crossing the small stream flowing from the spring. You descend on switchbacks through a forest dominated by mountain hemlock mixed with occasional western white pines. Where the grade lessens and you cross an avalanche zone with stunted trees, Fairview Dome dominates the view to the northwest. A second descent through a drier forest, this one dominated by lodgepole pine, brings you to a junction, just south of Hwy. 120, where a large map of the area is posted [8580' – 2.4/2.4]. Continuing straight ahead would bring you to the Cathedral Lakes parking area and a (free) Tuolumne Meadows shuttlebus stop, while the JMT continues east on a trail that roughly parallels the highway. The trail almost immediately crosses Budd Creek on a footbridge and you stroll through open lodgepole forest to reach another junction [8630' – 0.9/3.3]. At this junction, the official JMT (and therefore the route described here) heads north through Tuolumne Meadows and

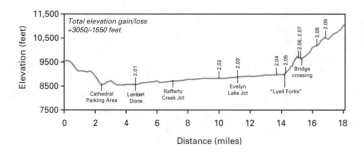

past the historic Parsons Lodge. However, many hikers opt to continue east on the trail paralleling Hwy. 120, a more direct route to the Tuolumne Meadows campground and beyond. If you choose the latter, head due east, ignoring all junctions: past the Elizabeth Lake junction (turning north here leads you into the campground), past the campground, continuing for approximately 2.3 miles through an open lodgepole forest until you rejoin the JMT just after it has crossed the Lyell Forks bridges.

Before you continue, a little Tuolumne Meadows orientation: Tuolumne Meadows amenities exist along the 1.5-mile east-west Hwy. 120 corridor beginning where the two possible routes diverge. From west to east, you will encounter a visitor center with an excellent bookstore and natural history displays, a small mountaineering store, the Tuolumne Meadows Grill, the grocery store, and the campground, the only legal camping from the lower Cathedral Lake until you are 4 miles up Lyell Canyon. The Tuolumne Meadows campground has a section

Location	Elevation	Distance from Previous Point	Cumulative Distance	UTM Coordinates
Mariposa-Tuolumne County Line	9570	—	0	11S 287795E 4192140N
Cathedral Lakes Parking Area junction	8580	2.4	2.4	11S 290450E 4194131N
Western merge with alternate route	8630	0.9	3.3	11S 291490E 4193887N
Parsons Lodge junction	8565	0.6	3.9	11S 291899E 4194771N
Lembert Dome parking area	8585	0.7	4.6	11S 293124E 4194586N
Tuolumne High Sierra Camp junction	8680	1.1	5.7	11S 294688E 4194424N
Eastern merge with alternate route	8670	0.6	6.3	11S 294824E 4193625N
Rafferty Creek junction	8720	0.7	7.0	11S 295739E 4193385N
Evelyn Lake junction	8900	4.2	11.2	11S 299489E 4188820N
Start of climb from Lyell Canyon (Lyell Forks)	9000	3.0	14.2	11S 300932E 4184713N
Bridge across Lyell Forks of the Tuolumne	9650	1.1	15.3	11S 300860E 4183344N
Wade across the Lyell Forks of the Tuolumne	10,185	1.0	16.3	11S 301333E 4182247N
Donohue Pass	11,060	1.8	18.1	11S 302007E 4181469N

SEE MAP 12

of walk-in campgrounds reserved for backpackers: These are due south of the Dana Campfire Circle and toward the eastern end of the campground, cost $5 per person, and allow only a one-night stay. Farther east, along a spur road, is first the wilderness permit station, and then, after a mile, the Tuolumne Meadows Lodge, where showers are available during the middle of the day. Meals and lodging are also available but must be reserved well in advance.

To follow the official, and certainly more scenic, JMT route, turn north (left) at the previously described junction. The trail shortly passes a junction to the visitor center and then reaches Hwy. 120. Cross the road and enter the wide-open, flower-filled Tuolumne Meadows, following the metal sign to Parsons Lodge. As the trail cuts north across the meadows, stop frequently and stare in all directions, enjoying the landscape of nearby domes, Unicorn and Cathedral peaks, and the large, red, rounded peaks to the east, Mt. Dana and Mt. Gibbs. Pothole Dome, to the west, and Lembert Dome, to the east, are good examples of roches moutonées. These formed as a glacier flowed up and over their tops. The ascending side is smooth and gentle, while the glacier plucked large chunks of rock on the downhill side, creating a jagged, steep topography. You may also note the young lodgepole pines encroaching on the meadows. Researchers have several hypotheses for their relentless invasion but have not yet reached a consensus on the cause. You cross the Tuolumne River on a footbridge below some buildings, Parsons Lodge and McCauley Cabin, at which you should stop and take a look [8565' – 0.6/3.9]. The Sierra Club built Parsons Lodge in 1915 as a mountain meeting room, and it is filled with written and photographic tales of historical Tuolumne. From Parsons Lodge, your path heads past the Soda Springs, where early tourists came to sample the soda water and relax. This was one of John Muir's favorite "hangouts" in Tuolumne, and where he conceived the idea of establishing Yosemite National Park. When you are ready to continue, the ever-present carved metal trail signs keep you headed eastward through the meadow, now on the route of the original Hwy. 120.

As you head east toward the steep granite face of Lembert Dome, take some time to read the informative signs along the road, describing both the human and natural history of the area. Shortly before the dome, you circumvent a gate that bars vehicular traffic and pass a spur road to the local stables. Keeping to the road, you pass below the dome and through its parking lot to reach the highway [8585' – 0.7/4.6]. The summit of Lembert Dome provides a 360-degree vista of the Tuolumne Meadows area; if you have a few hours, follow the trail northeast from

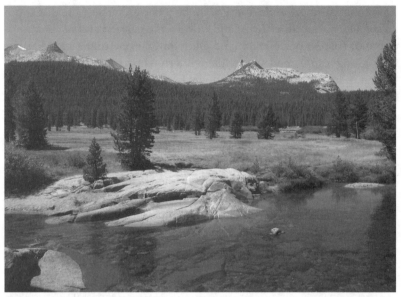

Tuolumne Meadows with Unicorn and Cathedral peaks in the background

the parking lot (see Appendix E). Cross the highway again, and pick up a wide dirt track to a large parking lot and the wilderness permit station, where rangers can both dispense wilderness permits and answer questions you pose regarding conditions. But please note that they are permitted only to dispense the most recent factual information available to them, and not to offer advice. This is often a source of frustration to both them and hikers. Your route now parallels the road to the Tuolumne Meadows Lodge. Shortly after you pass another large backpacker's parking lot, you curve southeast toward the Dana Fork of the Tuolumne River. Pass a signed spur trail to the Tuolumne Meadows Lodge (also known as the Tuolumne Meadows High Sierra Camp; 8680' – 1.1/5.7], cross the Dana Fork on a footbridge, and quickly reach a junction with a trail headed northeast to Gaylor Lakes. Staying on the JMT, you curve south and leave the Dana Fork drainage. Before long, the trail exits the dry lodgepole forest and reaches the Lyell Forks of the Tuolumne River. Cross the river on a pair of bridges, and look into the water at the exquisitely carved granite—smooth slabs and deep holes, dangerous if the water is high and perfect for a cold dip later in the season. In a few more steps, you re-enter forest and reach the junction where the official JMT reconnects with the route skirting the southern edge of the meadows [8670' – 0.6/6.3].

SEE MAP 12

As you leave Tuolumne Meadows, you no longer have to worry about heading in the correct direction at the junctions you had been encountering every few minutes and can once again focus on the beautiful scenery. Although you can't see it from the trail, you are paralleling the Lyell Forks eastward, passing alternately through sections of lodgepole forest with little ground cover and through small meadows. Although these openings appear grass-covered, many are inhabited by a group of related species, sedges, whose flowers are in small, dark heads. Sometimes individual plants appear as circles, where they have grown outward over many years. A common species here, and in many other meadows, is Parish's yampah, a member of the carrot family, with three linear leaf-lobes and a broad head of minute white flowers. Two species of pussytoes are also abundant at the meadow edges. These species form extensive mats, have small, elongate, and quite fuzzy leaves and flowers that resemble tiny tufts of fuzz. Rosy pussytoes' flowers have a pinkish tinge, while others, such as flat-topped pussytoes, are white. These areas are also a favorite haunt of the mule deer. The bucks are tame and sport large antlers in the sanctuary provided by the national park boundaries. Cassin's finches, with a red head and streaked pinkish back, and red crossbills, somewhat larger and with the eponymous crossed beak, are both present in this forest. Your next junction is with the Rafferty Creek Trail [8720' – 0.7/7.0], which heads south to Vogelsang High Sierra Camp.

In another 0.7 mile, the trail and the river curve south-southeast, and the two converge; the trail often runs in the meadow lining the river. You get to enjoy this idyllic scene for the next many miles: The walls of Lyell Canyon rise steeply on either side; the unbelievably clear and often deep, aqua-green waters of the Lyell Forks meander down the middle of the canyon; and flower-filled meadows line the edges of the stream. If you are lucky, you will spot a belted kingfisher, with its shrill, cackling call, diving into the water to fish. Your only job is not to disturb the scene for the next party: Be sure to stay on the trail and not trespass into the meadow each time the track becomes a bit deeper or muddier. Two of the flower species you will see throughout Lyell Canyon are the Sierra penstemon, with a circular arrangement of 2–centimeter-long, skinny, tubular, purple flowers, and little elephant's head, with an elongated head of 0.5-centimeter long, lavender flowers. If you look at an individual flower upside down, you can see the elephant's ears and trunk. Both are present in nearly every high elevation wet meadow in the Sierra, and the Sierra penstemon also thrives in drier environments.

SEE MAP 12

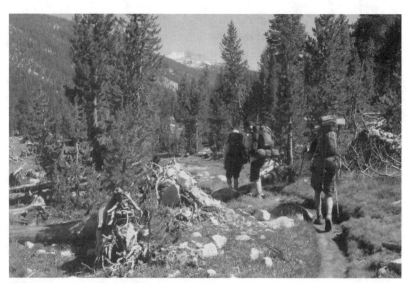

Walking past avalanche debris in Lyell Canyon

Camping is not allowed in Lyell Canyon until you are 4 miles beyond Tuolumne Meadows, a position approximately marked by a large avalanche path visible on the east canyon wall. While you can always find a few small campsites to the edge of the meadow, the first major camping area is at the junction with the trail to Ireland and Evelyn lakes [8900' – 4.2/11.2], where there are many campsites just to the northwest of the trail junction. Ireland Creek is easy to wade, or you can work your way across a series of logs to the west of the trail that are often half submerged during high flow. Still with negligible elevation gain, the JMT continues up Lyell Canyon, beneath imposing Potter Point. Where the trail diverges slightly from the river, there are a few campsites. Eventually, you reach an area where the river branches, at the "Lyell Forks," and soon thereafter you begin to climb out of Lyell Canyon [9000' – 3.0/14.2]. There are additional campsites just at the start of the climb.

From Lyell Forks base camp, you begin to climb a series of exposed switchbacks, mostly across a slope strewn with avalanche debris. One of the common shrubs on these disturbed slopes is mountain red elderberry, distinguished by its large leaves, in clusters of seven: By midsummer, the berries are a favorite food source for wildlife. As you continue climbing, you leave the lodgepole forests that fringe Lyell Canyon and enter stands dominated by mountain hemlocks. The switchbacks end at a forested bench with many campsites. The trail then crosses the

SEE MAP 12

Lyell Forks [9650' – 1.1/15.3] on a footbridge before resuming its ascent through mixed hemlock and lodgepole forest. The slope next lessens at a small lake [10,185' – 1.0/16.3], fringed by a charming timberline meadow and scattered stands of whitebark pines, the most common timberline species throughout the Sierra; its needles are in clusters of five, which easily distinguishes it from the oft-intermixed lodgepoles. There are a few good campsites and many less-ideal sites used by the latecomers. If you choose to spend the night here, you will begin your morning with a chilly wade across the lake near its outlet, followed by a steep climb up a slope west of the small lake. Numerous trickles cross this slope and the vegetation is lush, until you suddenly level out to the side of a sandy knob. You next drop down to a second stream crossing. There are a few small, sandy tent sites in the area, used mainly by climbers headed to the summit of Mt. Lyell, the imposing 13,114-foot peak to the south that is Yosemite's highest. The snowfield you see is the largest glacier visible from the JMT. Notably, all current glaciers in the Sierra Nevada formed during the Little Ice Age, a cold period that began 700 years ago. The much larger Pleistocene glaciers had completely disappeared in the interim. The views of Mt. Lyell continue to improve as you begin the final climb to Donohue Pass. Alongside rocks, near seasonal streams, you may see the white mountain heather, one of John Muir's favorite flowers. These flowers are shaped like little white bells with red caps and can occur in large masses. Also present is the red mountain heather, with more open, red-pink flowers and longer, needle-shaped leaves. Both form mats alongside rocks, although the red heather grows down to lower elevations, has a range that extends farther south in the Sierra, and is much more abundant. The ascent continues on granite slabs and along sandy passageways, delineating fractures in the granite. Before long, you emerge on the summit of tarn-dotted Donohue Pass [11,060' – 1.8/18.1]. If you wish to climb still higher, a side trip up Donohue Peak is recommended (see Appendix E).

SEE MAPS 11–12

SECTION 3.

Donohue Pass to
Island Pass—Rush Creek

onohue Pass delineates the boundary between Yosemite National Park and Ansel Adams Wilderness. To the south you can see
Mammoth Mountain and the Mammoth Crest, country you will traverse over the coming days. The next 4.9-mile leg to the top of Island
Pass is the only section of the JMT that is east of the Sierra Crest: Rush
Creek drains into Mono Lake, the famous Great Basin salt lake with
no outlet. You descend switchbacks, enjoying the view of the alpine,
meadow-covered, granite basin with abundant glacial erratics—large
boulders scattered across the landscape where they were "dumped"
by a glacier. The abundance of heath vegetation is an indication of just
how wet this area is: dwarf bilberry, white heather, red heather, and
bog kalmia, which has flowers quite similar to red heather, but forming
upright carpets in flat, marshy areas and sporting larger leaves. There
are also the diminutive arctic willows crawling along the ground, most
easily identifiable if covered by the white fuzz that accompanies their

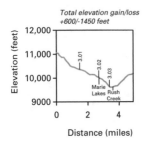

SEE MAP 11

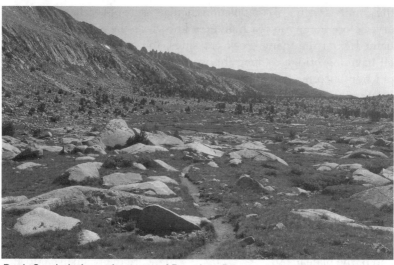

Rush Creek drainage just east of Donohue Pass

flowers. Endless small creek crossings may slow your progress in early season, and the marshy, vegetated ground is mostly too wet and fragile for camping; only a few drier hummocks, denoted by stunted white-bark pines, offer dry, legal, and certainly worthwhile campsites; seek out sandy, previously used sites.

Your descent crosses increasingly forested terrain, and before long you reach the roaring torrent of Rush Creek. A new log bridge allows you to cross the flow safely, and just across the stream, you reach the junction with the Marie Lakes Trail [10,040' – 2.7/2.7], where there are a couple of campsites. As you continue your switchbacking descent, you may notice the granite getting darker: You are approaching the boundary between granitic and metamorphosed volcanic rocks, and

Location	Elevation	Distance from Previous Point	Cumulative Distance	UTM Coordinates
Donohue Pass	11,060	—	0	11S 302007E 4181469N
Marie Lakes junction	10,040	2.7	2.7	11S 304471E 4180124N
Rush Creek junction	9640	0.9	3.6	11S 305257E 4179482N
Davis Lakes junction	9680	0.3	3.9	11S 305502E 4179278N
Island Pass	10,205	1.0	4.9	11S 306699E 4178705N

SEE MAP 11

the granite's chemical composition changes as it approaches the boundary. Before long, you reach an area known as the Rush Creek Forks, named from the many creek crossings, the more difficult of which all have log bridges. Along the way, you pass the Rush Creek Trail junction, incorrectly marked about 0.15 mile to the north of its actual location on the USGS topo maps [9640' – 0.9/3.6]. You also pass the Davis Lakes junction [9680' – 0.3/3.9] and begin the climb to Island Pass. The north-facing climb is through dry lodgepole forest with little ground cover, although it's certainly not bare. Pussytoes, which have small balls of pink flowers on short stalks, is one species that tolerates such inhospitable conditions. Its long, skinny, dark green, and slightly succulent leaves hug the ground. The rock here is a mixture of various meta-volcanics, and it will be many miles before you see granite again. Shortly, the climb ends amongst dry meadows and many marshy tarns atop Island Pass. The unmarked high point is toward the northern end of the plateau [10,205' – 1.0/4.9]. There are many small campsites amongst the ponds—take a look around.

SEE MAP 11

SECTION 4.

Island Pass to Madera-Fresno County Line—Middle Fork of the San Joaquin River

From now until the summit of Mt. Whitney, the JMT is again on the west side of the crest: All water drains into the San Joaquin Valley. For more than 85 miles, you will be in the drainage of the San Joaquin River, whose waters eventually flow into the San Francisco Bay. You will be first descending the main Middle Fork drainage, then ascending the Fish Creek drainage, crossing Mono Creek, Bear Creek, and finally entering the main South Fork drainage that you follow to Muir Pass. But of more interest to you now is the sweeping view of the dark Ritter Range, of which, Banner Peak, the northernmost peak, stands out most prominently. You descend dry slopes toward Thousand Island Lake, whose surface is dotted with dozens of rocky islets. Although dry, the volcanic soils sport an amazing diversity of wildflowers—including a

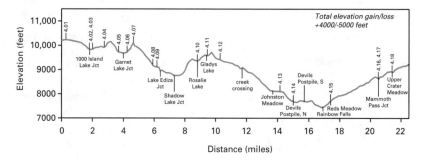

SEE MAP 11

patch of periwinkle-colored western blue flax, a species you will not see again until you ascend the slopes of Mt. Whitney, and large masses of pretty faces, pale yellow, six-petal flowers related to lilies. Bright blue mountain bluebirds are commonly seen on these bare slopes, perched on snags between insect-catching forays. As the descent levels out, you reach a junction with a trail that leads around the lake's northwest shore, where there are many camping options. Note that camping is prohibited within a quarter mile of the lake's outlet. Views of Banner Peak

Location	Elevation	Distance from Previous Point	Cumulative Distance	UTM Coordinates
Island Pass	10,205	—	0	11S 306699E 4178705N
Thousand Island Lake junction	9830	1.8	1.8	11S 308736E 4177715N
Garnet Lake junction	9680	2.2	4.0	11S 310475E 4176159N
Lake Ediza junction	9000	2.4	6.4	11S 311088E 4173423N
Shadow Lake junction	8760	0.9	7.3	11S 311695E 4173764N
Rosalie Lake outlet	9350	1.5	8.8	11S 313028E 4173139N
Gladys Lake	9575	0.6	9.4	11S 313189E 4172430N
Trinity Lakes outlet crossing	9045	2.3	11.7	11S 314721E 4170195N
Johnston Meadow	8120	2.0	13.7	11S 314827E 4168538N
Beck Lakes junction	8090	0.6	14.3	11S 315353E 4167777N
Northern Devils Postpile junction	7685	0.7	15.0	11S 315747E 4166939N
Southern Devils Postpile junction	7710	0.7	15.7	11S 315855E 4165917N
Rainbow Falls junction	7475	1.2	16.9	11S 316244E 4164846N
Reds Meadow junction	7715	0.5	17.4	11S 316900E 4164357N
Crater Creek crossing at Red Cones	8645	3.1	20.5	11S 318338E 4162253N
Mammoth Pass junction in Upper Crater Meadow	8915	0.9	21.4	11S 319252E 4161498N
Madera-Fresno County Line	9220	1.1	22.5	11S 319953E 4160145N

SEE MAP 11

over Thousand Island Lake are irresistible for photographers and were memorialized in many of Ansel Adams' most famous photographs—how appropriate that this area is now part of his namesake wilderness. A few more steps bring you to a junction where the JMT and the Pacific Crest Trail (PCT), which have been one and the same since Tuolumne Meadows, diverge for several miles [9830' – 1.8/1.8].

You head southeast on a footbridge over the outlet of Thousand Island Lake, noting additional campsites on the bluff to the southwest of the lake, and make a moderate climb past pretty Emerald Lake, whose western shore is closed to camping. You continue upward to Ruby Lake, surrounded on the west by impressive walls, and to the northeast by enormous mats of manzanita. There are small campsites near the outlet, beneath mountain hemlock cover. The JMT climbs again, to the ridgetop above Ruby Lake, before descending on rocky switchbacks to beautiful, windy Garnet Lake, a smaller version of Thousand Island Lake, which is likewise dotted with islets. Note that, as for Thousand Island Lake, camping is prohibited within a quarter mile of Garnet Lake's outlet. Fortunately, near the bottom of the switchbacks, you find a junction with a use trail that leads to campsites on Garnet's northwest shore; the sites get better the farther you go toward Garnet's head. While only Banner Peak was visible from Thousand Island Lake, both Mt. Ritter and Banner Peak are now prominent. You trace Garnet's north shore briefly, passing large patches of red heather, cross its outlet on a footbridge, and immediately pass a junction with a rough trail that descends northeast into the canyon of the Middle Fork of the San Joaquin River [9680' – 2.2/4.0].

Now the JMT traces Garnet's south shore briefly, passing through wet streamside vegetation that includes the bright red great red paintbrush. Paintbrushes have elongated heads of very narrow, tubular, beaked flowers, and the great red paintbrush is the tallest of the many Sierra species. It is also the only one to prefer stream banks and seeps. You pass one more campsite perched on a small flat to the side of the lake before turning southeast to climb steeply up the ridge south of Garnet Lake. Halfway up, near a giant mountain hemlock, are tufts of bell-shaped, (light) pink heuchera emerging from cracks in the rock. At a saddle atop the ridge, there are few mediocre tent sites and a swimming-pool-sized pond that warms up enough by midsummer for pleasant bathing.

You now begin a 1100-foot descent, past a small meadow and through a tiny canyon with mixed lodgepole pine and mountain hemlock cover. The two-tone needles of the latter always stand out: The

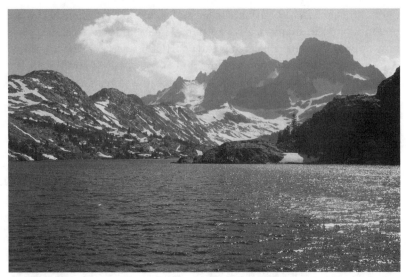

Garnet Lake with Mt. Ritter and Banner Peak in the background

young needles are a much brighter green than the old foliage. A few western white pines, with their larger cones, are also present. Before long, you emerge on a dry knob with majestic western juniper, an understory of manzanita, and an excellent view of the Minarets, the skyline of spires to the south of Mt. Ritter. Shortly after you re-enter the forest, you converge with a tributary of Shadow Creek and pass shady flats with good campsites. Soon you reach a T-junction: A right turn takes you to Ediza Lake, while the JMT turns east (left) to Shadow Lake and Agnew Meadows [9000' – 2.4/6.4].

You alternately descend through lodgepole forest and across open, slabby knobs, still composed of meta-volcanic rock. The fast-flowing stream is a good location to spot an American dipper, also known as a water ouzel—a round, grayish bird that can often be seen diving in and out of rapids in search of insects; its constantly bending knees confirm its identity. Along the JMT, camping is prohibited between the previously described junction and Shadow Lake, 0.9 mile to the east. If this regulation is relaxed in the future, please still consider camping outside of this very high-use corridor; this is a favorite destination for weekend hikers. At the Shadow Lake inlet, you reach another junction: Straight ahead takes you down to the Middle Fork of the San Joaquin River and out to Agnew Meadows, while the JMT turns south (right) across a handsome footbridge [8760' – 0.9/7.3].

SEE MAP 11

The elevation profile certainly indicates there is a long climb ahead, but do not be too discouraged, as the switchbacks are well-graded and the dense hemlock forest will provide nearly continuous shade. A little more than 650 feet later, you reach a small saddle and briefly emerge from the forest, before descending to shady Rosalie Lake. There are mountain hemlocks overhead and poisonous western Labrador tea underfoot as you approach a logjam across the outlet [9350' – 1.5/8.8]. The latter resembles an azalea, and indeed the two are in the same family. There are some nice campsites nearby.

You skirt Rosalie's north and east shores before climbing a little and then dipping down to mountain hemlock-fringed Gladys Lake [9575' – 0.6/9.4], which also has a number of good campsites. After passing Gladys Lake, the JMT rolls over a little saddle and begins a long, gradual descent of Volcanic Ridge, still under mountain hemlocks, western white pines, and a few lodgepole pines. You pass the attractive, marshy Trinity Lakes, a series of shallow ponds strung out along the trail. If you are willing to walk a few hundred feet to water, there are many sandy campsites on the west side of the trail, but also keep your eyes peeled for campsites closer to water. The JMT skirts lower Trinity Lake and shortly crosses the Trinity Lakes outlet [9045' – 2.3/11.7], with a colorful display of wildflowers, including crimson columbine, with bright, red-orange flowers that point upright and five long spurs that dangle behind. This forest is lower elevation than many along the JMT and is filled with birdlife: Keep your ears open for a black-backed woodpecker whacking on a dead tree or a northern goshawk screeching as it flies through the forest.

Both the angle of the slope and the angle of your descent now increase, the slope becomes drier, and the vegetation changes. For the first time since Sunrise Creek, you encounter red fir, mixed in with continued western white pines and a few lodgepole pines. Most of your descent is on a dry and sandy pumice slope, with red-colored Anderson's thistles and aromatic pennyroyal, a mint, but occasionally you cross a small seep and encounter a wetter plant community. Just north of Johnston Meadow, you reach a T-junction with a trail that goes northwest to Minaret Lake, while the JMT heads southeast toward Devils Postpile [8120' – 2.0/13.7]. Across the trail are boggy Johnston Meadow and little Johnston Lake.

The JMT continues descending over loose pumice, passing a few campsites, to a crossing of Minaret Creek on a log bridge. (This enticing, pebble-bottomed creek would be a wonderful place to cool your feet.) You shortly pass a junction with a trail west to Beck Lakes [8090'

– 0.6/14.3] and continue down a dry, open, pumice slope to a large X-junction just inside the boundary of Devils Postpile National Monument [7685' – 0.7/15.0]. At this point, the PCT, coming in from the northeast, rejoins the JMT.

Although the JMT continues along the southwestern branch of the X, if you have not previously visited Devils Postpile, I recommend a detour to this geologic attraction, since the JMT provides only fleeting and distant glances of the structure. Others may take the junction to Devils Postpile to find camping for the night or to access Mammoth Lakes. There are campgrounds at both Devils Postpile and near the Reds Meadow Resort, a short distance to the south, although only at Reds Meadow are there showers and sites specially reserved for backpackers. Both locations also provide access to the shuttle bus, which runs every 30 minutes midseason and travels to the Mammoth Mountain ski area, your "gateway" to the town of Mammoth Lakes.

To reach Devils Postpile, take the southeast-trending fork down to the riverbank, where you soon find a bridge. Cross the bridge and continue south to a short, sign-posted loop around the postpile. A bit of geologic background: Devils Postpile formed less than 100,000 years ago, following an eruption of basaltic magma. Slow, even cooling conditions and magma with a consistent chemical composition throughout allowed the hexagonal columns to form. Because of the topography, an unusually deep flow of magma accumulated, such that the interior was well-insulated and cooled slowly and evenly. As magma cools, it contracts and hence must fracture. Physics dictates that fractures 120 degrees apart most efficiently release building stress, leading to hexagonal columns. Devils Postpile is one of the world's tallest and most nearly perfect examples of columnar basalt. Be sure to walk around the loop, which takes you both to the top of the formation, where glacially polished tops of columns are exposed, and to the base of the formation, where you can gaze up at the columns and gawk at the talus field of hexagonal-shaped rocks. From the southern end of this short loop, follow the trail that leads to Rainbow Falls. This trail intersects the JMT near the Reds Meadow Resort: At 7460 feet, near the riverbank, you reach a junction, where you turn southeast (left) onto the JMT.

To bypass Devils Postpile, take the upper, south-trending fork and climb gently up a dusty track across a steep, pumice slope. With the exception of one knob, the postpiles are hidden from view. You pass a second X-junction, where another trail from Devils Postpile crosses the JMT and heads southwest toward King Creek [7710' – 0.7/15.7]. The JMT continues to the southeast. Shortly after this junction, you

SEE MAP 10

enter a burn area, the result of a large, lightning-caused forest fire in 1992, named the Rainbow Fire. The dusty pumice substrate might be even less appealing without forest cover, but the open slopes display abundant bird life, including yellow-rumped warblers, mountain blue-birds, and swallows, as well as a community of plants that only thrive following burns. You will walk past abundant Sierra gooseberries with 1–centimeter-wide, spiny (but otherwise tasty) berries; mountain whitethorn, a shrub with intimidating thorns and small, blue-green leaves; and scarlet penstemon, with its stalk full of bright red, tubular flowers. Shortly, you cross the Middle Fork of the San Joaquin on a footbridge and almost immediately reach a junction, where those hav-ing detoured to Devils Postpile will rejoin the JMT [7475' – 1.2/16.9]. From this point, you can also detour south to Rainbow Falls if you have the time and energy.

From this junction, the JMT leaves Devils Postpile National Monu-ment and heads east toward Reds Meadow. Over the next half mile, you will pass three more junctions. The third [7715' – 0.5/17.4] pro-vides the most efficient access to the Reds Meadow Resort, where you may have a food parcel to retrieve, wish to eat at the café, fill your water bottles, buy additional supplies, or find a campground for the night (see Appendix C for details). Continuing on the JMT, you ascend yet another pumice trail, still in the area denuded by the Rainbow Fire. If you find yourself annoyed by its dusty nature, stop and appreciate how soft it is underfoot! As before, the wildflower displays can be astonish-ing and the aerial antics of the abundant swallows engaging. And as you stare at the thick, spiny shrubs on either side of the trail, you'll be thankful to be on a maintained trail. Camping is impractical along this stretch of the JMT due to the dense undergrowth, and you must reach Crater Creek by nightfall. As you climb, you first cross four branches of Boundary Creek and slowly, as the slope becomes steeper, enter ar-eas with more standing trees—Jeffrey pines, western junipers, western white pines, and white firs. In the distance, you can see the outline of the two Red Cones. Many switchbacks later, you find yourself at the base of the northern Red Cone, at a little-used and poorly marked junction with a trail northeast to Mammoth Pass [8645' – 3.1/20.5]. Just beyond this point, you cross Crater Creek on a fallen log. Along the stream banks, a short distance below the crossing, a few, mostly collapsed, lava tubes are visible. There are several campsites on the south side of Crater Creek and one a short distance up the northern Red Cone.

An ascent of one (or both) of the Red Cones is highly recommend-ed (see Appendix E). The vista from the summit not only lets you gaze

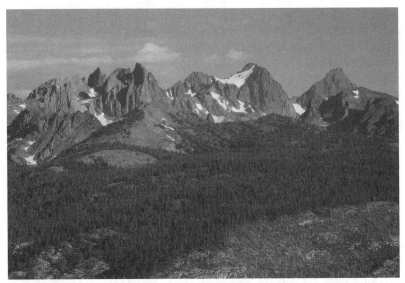

The Minarets, Mt. Ritter, and Banner Peak viewed from atop the Red Cones

over the country you've covered since Donohue Pass, but you also get a close-up view of Mammoth Mountain. A bit of geologic history: The volcanic activity of the last 3 million years formed the pumice deposits you have walked over and will continue to walk over. About 760,000 years ago, an enormous eruption formed Long Valley Caldera, a bit east of the Sierra, depositing ash as far east as Nebraska. At 220,000 years, Mammoth Mountain, a dormant volcano, is a more recent addition. These events are separate from the much older volcanic events that led to the formation of the Ritter Range. Those dark rocks likely resulted from a catastrophic caldera collapse 100 million years ago, and have since been metamorphosed during the tectonic events that led to the emplacement of the underlying granite. Today Mammoth Mountain is best known as an enormous ski area that receives enormous quantities of snow. This is no coincidence, as the passes crossing the Sierra Crest in this vicinity are the lowest for a great distance north and south, allowing storms that are elsewhere blocked by tall mountains to funnel straight to the slopes of Mammoth. Its founder, who had previously worked as a snow surveyor, had done his homework.

From Crater Creek, you continue south up a small ravine, cross Crater Creek again, and emerge at lovely Upper Crater Meadow. Abundant wet meadow wildflowers can be seen here, including several species forming mats along the ground, such as carpet clover, which has

SEE MAPS 9–10

small, white flowers, and primrose monkeyflower, which has single, yellow, tubular flowers attached atop 2- to 4-inch stalks. It is always identifiable by its light green leaves pressed flat to the ground and long hairs that hold the morning dew and cause the plants to glow in the sun. As you continue south along the JMT, these species will become familiar faces in wet alpine meadows or at the borders of little seeps. Campsites can be found in the forested fringes around the meadow. Several tracks leave the meadow, all headed toward Mammoth Pass. The southernmost of these tracks is the main one [8915' – 0.9/21.4].

From Upper Crater Meadow, the JMT crunches south-southeast over pumice, crossing a small fork of Crater Creek, and then crossing Crater Creek itself again. This gradual ascent ends approximately 0.2 mile after the last creek crossing, atop a sandy saddle and unlikely drainage divide. This point, the Madera-Fresno County Line, marks the boundary between the main Middle Fork of the San Joaquin drainage and Fish Creek [9220' – 1.1/22.5].

SEE MAPS 9–10

SECTION 5.

Madera-Fresno County Line to Silver Pass—Fish Creek Fork of the Middle Fork of the San Joaquin River

From the drainage divide, the JMT continues through open lodgepole forest. It drops a little, passes an indistinct and unmarked junction with a lateral up Deer Creek, and then fords Deer Creek [9100' – 0.9/0.9], to either side of which are a number of campsites frequented by stock parties. Fill your water bottles at Deer Creek, for the next reliable water is at Duck Creek, nearly 6 miles away. To many, the next section is among the most monotonous on the JMT: Until you approach the Duck Pass junction, the vegetation and views change little. But pay close attention to a change in rock type, as you are still on pumice substrate initially, but will transition to granite as you climb gradually along the north wall of Cascade Valley. At first, the forest contains a mixture of

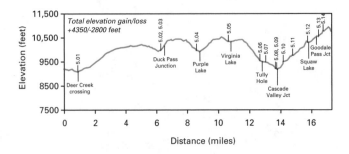

SEE MAP 9

lodgepole and western white pine, but the western white pines disappear before long, as only lodgepole pines can survive under the dry conditions dictated by the southern exposure and coarse volcanic soils. The ground, likewise, is nearly bare—most notable are a few species in the mustard family, whose flowers are distinguished by a four-petal arrangement resembling a cross: western wallflower, with its heads of many yellow flowers on a tall stalk, and several types of rock cress, with small, white to purple flowers on a slightly shorter stem. By mid-season, most individual plants no longer have flowers and are instead decorated by long seedpods; species of rock cress are distinguished by the width of the pods and whether they are upright or drooping. Occasionally, a rocky slope sports a few shrubs, including mountain sagebrush, manzanita, and a relative of oaks, bush chinquapin, whose leaf undersides are gold-colored. Openings in the forest provide occasional glimpses south to the Silver Divide. Among the many birds you are likely to see in this area are the red-breasted nuthatches, circling down a tree trunk in search of insects, and "honking" like a truck backing up; the ubiquitous dark-eyed junco, a large sparrow with a dark head and streaks of white on its tail; and blue grouse. Toward the end of this long, ascending traverse, you cross onto granite, at last leaving the pumice behind. After a few days of the foot-pounding granite cobble

Location	Elevation	Distance from Previous Point	Cumulative Distance	UTM Coordinates
Madera-Fresno County Line	9220	—	0	11S 319953E 4160145N
Deer Creek crossing	9100	0.9	0.9	11S 320455E 4159144N
Duck Pass junction	10,170	5.6	6.5	11S 326105E 4156217N
Purple Lake outlet	9925	2.3	8.8	11S 327825E 4154989N
Lake Virginia inlet	10,338	2.0	10.8	11S 329261E 4153679N
Tully Hole junction	9520	2.0	12.8	11S 329943E 4152061N
Cascade Creek junction	9190	1.0	13.8	11S 329182E 4150922N
Squaw Lake outlet	10,300	2.0	15.8	11S 329950E 4149412N
Goodale Pass junction	10,530	0.5	16.3	11S 329472E 4149131N
Silver Pass	10,750	1.0	17.3	11S 330017E 4148322N

SEE MAP 9

and gravel, you might even begin to miss the dusty but soft, pumice sand. Eventually, you make an easy descent into the valley of Duck Creek, where a handful of small campsites are clustered among granite slabs near the western side of the crossing. Follow the western creek bank downstream to find additional sites. The ford across Duck Creek is not dangerous, but under high water it is a likely wade. A little beyond the creek, the JMT begins a switchbacking climb past a junction with a trail to Duck Lake and Duck Pass [10,170' – 5.6/6.5].

From the junction, your ascent continues out of the Duck Creek valley and back around to a southern exposure. Here, there are few trees, and you have a beautiful view of the walls of glaciated Cascade Valley and southeast toward Mt. Abbot, a peak on the Sierra Crest. Although it is dry, many flowers dot the granite soil. You may have seen two earlier: the wavy-leaved paintbrush and shaggy hawkweed. The paintbrush, a dominant species on all dry slopes, sports a dense head of red-orange tubular flowers and is distinguished from the many other paintbrushes by its wavy-margined leaves. The hawksweed has small yellow flowers that look like miniature dandelions, and its leaves are covered in long white hairs. Pennyroyal and mountain pride pentstemon are also common here. Before long, you reach a use trail that leads north to campsites on the west shore of beautiful Purple Lake. The JMT continues toward Purple Lake's outlet, passing a junction that leads down into Cascade Valley [9925' – 2.3/8.8]. In the past, the ford across the outlet stream could be difficult, but a new bridge makes for an easy crossing. Camping is prohibited within 300 feet of the outlet.

Now the JMT makes a dry, switchbacking climb to the ridge east of Purple Lake, before leveling out as you approach a wide saddle. Near the summit, spreading carpets of Sierra arnica grace some of the slopes. These large yellow flowers, related to sunflowers, appear sporadically in open lodgepole forests. Nearer the saddle is a community of dry-site subalpine and alpine species. Large patches of long-stemmed, five-petal white flowers with "mousetail" like stalks of leaves may stand out—mousetail ivesia. Steep walls and talus fields greet you at the summit, the first time you have encountered such landscape on your southward journey. The pile of rock just to the south of the trail is not a moraine, but a rock glacier, a large mound of talus, likely with ice in its core and slowly moving downslope. The ice at the center of rock glaciers may be much older than that in the Sierra's ice glaciers, possibly providing a longer climatic record for the Sierra—if only there were an easy way to core into it. As you travel farther south, these will become a common feature.

SEE MAP 9

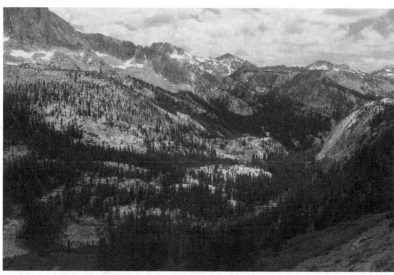

Tully Hole and Cascade Valley

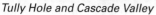

You now descend to Lake Virginia [10,338' – 2.0/10.8], a lovely, large subalpine lake with open views to the south and colorful meadows along its northern shore. Particularly striking are two more species of paintbrush to add to your growing palette, the purple Lemmon's paintbrush and the red and yellow mountain paintbrush. Like the two species you have seen previously, these paintbrushes have dense heads of pointed tubular flowers, but only these two species of paintbrush occur in such enormous masses, coloring an entire meadow. There are campsites among scattered trees on the sandy knob to the northwest of the lake. As you leave the lake, stop in the first stand of lodgepole pines—this is a good place to see mountain chickadees, as the trees here have low branches where you may see the little birds, turned upside-down as they feed. You can always tell when these birds are nearby by their *chick-a-dee-dee* call; one higher, shorter note, followed by two lower, longer ones.

From Lake Virginia, the trail climbs gradually upward and curves southeast over a broad, sandy saddle before switchbacking down a steep, dry slope toward Tully Hole. The verdant meadow around Tully Hole and the lovely headwaters of the Fish Creek drainage look enticing from above—and since you are still above the mosquitoes, you can enjoy the view without the annoyance of the bugs below. As you descend the switchbacks, you will note that this seemingly desolate, dry, sandy slope is alive with an enormous diversity of flowers. Many are

SEE MAP 9

the species that have occurred on every dry slope you have traversed: shaggy hawkweed, scarlet penstemon, Anderson's thistles, pennyroyal, and the wavy-leaved paintbrush. Lower down the slope, you approach a few little streams and note the denser vegetation that grows where water is abundant. One beautiful wet-site plant is Coulter's daisy, a white daisy with many exquisitely narrow ray petals. Just past a large campsite used by pack groups, you reach Tully Hole and a junction with the trail that crosses Fish Creek to climb eastward up to McGee Pass [9520' – 2.0/12.8].

Meanwhile, the JMT descends Fish Creek's impressive west bank, passing beautiful sections of slab and deep swimming holes, as well as a few campsites. Before long, you emerge from the lodgepole forest onto a steep slope with picturesque western junipers, before descending to Fish Creek, which you cross on a steel footbridge. The three-petal, mostly white flowers of the Leichtlin's mariposa lily dot these slopes; *mariposa* is the Spanish word for butterfly, and the petals of many mariposa lilies indeed look like brightly colored wings. After the stream crossing, you enter the first diverse conifer forest since Crater Meadow. You pass one campsite shortly before a small creek crossing and a second on a knob just before the Cascade Valley junction [9190' – 1.0/13.8]. The trail junction, nestled among avalanche debris, is not always obviously marked, so make sure you take the left fork that begins the climb up to Silver Pass. This junction may be particularly confusing because many maps, including the USGS 7.5-minute topos, show the junction farther downstream. In fact, the trail goes straight up and does not cross the side drainage here.

The JMT turns southeast here and begins ascending toward Silver Pass along the east side of the creek. You are traveling through a dense hemlock and lodgepole forest. The thick tree cover feels odd in the Sierra, where you nearly always have a filtered view through the trees. Occasional benches to the west of the trail provide small campsites, ringed by heath vegetation: Labrador tea, dwarf bilberries, and red mountain heather are common in the understory. Black-eyed juncos and American robin, a species of thrush with a burnt red belly, are likely present around the tree bases. Around 9700 feet, you emerge from this magical forest and cross the creek twice, once at a lupine-covered crossing and shortly thereafter on a footbridge in front of a beautiful little marshy meadow. There is a campsite amongst open trees just southeast of the crossing.

As you resume your upward journey on a relatively steep trail, the forest becomes thinner and drier. You skirt around to the south-facing side of the ravine, noting only stunted trees and vegetation of dry, subalpine, granite slopes. Many of the species were also abundant at lower elevations, while others will become ever more common as you approach the higher passes to the south. At these elevations, Clark's nutcrackers, relatives of the jays, are common and noisy. These light grey and black birds feed on pine nuts and congregate from the upper elevation lodgepole forests to the timberline. More amazing is their natural history: They breed in March in the Sierra, so unless you are on skis, you will never see the young. They sustain themselves through the winter by eating from large stashes of whitebark pine nuts, buried on a diversity of slope aspects to ensure a continuous supply as the snow melts.

Alongside outcropping rock, you may note a succulent with small yellow star-like flowers, Sierra stonecrop. One of the common shrubs on this slope, small-leaved cream bush, boasts white, five-petal flowers on pinkish stems and small, serrate leaves. The trail levels out at small Squaw Lake, which is surrounded by alpine meadows and steep cliffs [10,300′ – 2.0/15.8]. A few sandy, exposed campsites are available to the northwest of its outlet. Camping here or along the next miles toward Silver Pass lets you absorb the alpine scenery for the first time since Donohue Pass. You cross the outlet on large solid rocks.

From Squaw Lake, you climb briefly and then level out at a junction with the trail from Goodale Pass [10,530′ – 0.5/16.3]. The JMT heads south-southeast to skirt dramatic Chief Lake. You are now just about at timberline, stunted whitebark pines still dot the landscape, but the ground cover is dominated by low-growing alpine species. Frosted buckwheat, a common species down into montane forests, forms large mats and is easily identified by its small, fuzzy leaves and ball-like heads of minute yellow flowers that turn red as they go to seed. There are a few sandy, exposed campsites amongst the tarns north of Chief Lake and also, when water is available, to the left side of the trail as you approach the pass. Through much of the season, there may be a small but quite steep snowbank as you ascend to a shoulder just before Silver Pass. The official pass (and drainage divide) is after you have descended the first two switchbacks [10,750′ – 1.0/17.3].

SEE MAP 8

SECTION 6.

Silver Pass to Selden Pass—Mono and Bear Creeks

Along these next miles of the JMT, you will travel the farthest from the Sierra Crest and often at lower elevations. Be sure to enjoy the expansive forests, as they will become more sparse as you head south and higher. But now you should enjoy the excellent view south, where you can observe much of your route to the top of Selden Pass. Seven Gables is one of the most dramatic peaks, and its sub-peak, to the west, has the seven namesake gables or ridges, running longitudinally down its north face. As you descend the sandy trail, note that the vegetation is different on the warmer, southern side of the pass. To the west is a small pothole lake with sapphire-blue water. As you approach the larger Silver Pass Lake, you walk alternately across stretches of alpine meadow and open, sandy flats. The latter are inhabited by Belding's ground squirrels, resembling miniature groundhogs in shape and in behavior as they stand upright and stare at you from their burrow entrances. The JMT curves eastward, away from Silver Pass Lake, but if

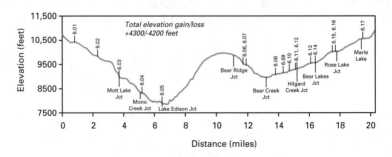

SEE MAP 8

you wish to camp here, you will find several sandy tent sites nestled among the lodgepole pines at the southeast end of the lake.

You then descend increasingly forested benches interspersed with openings surrounding granite slabs. Alongside outcropping rock, clusters of bright, rose-pink flowers on the shrub dense-flowered spiraea are likely to catch your attention. Before long, you pass several campsites under open lodgepole cover, and shortly afterward, ford Silver Pass Creek. The track now skirts the southwestern edge of a large meadow with a meandering stream, its edges lined by western bistort, with tall stalks and dense heads of small white flowers. This species slowly disappears from the meadow community as you continue south. As you round the next corner, the valley drops steeply in front of you and the vista opens up. Before you tackle the loose, rocky switchbacks, take a brief break to enjoy the waterfall and beautiful granite slabs to your left (east). Partway down the slope, the trail re-fords Silver Pass Creek. This can be a dangerous crossing because of the dashing cascades above and below you. With luck, though, there will be a series of well-placed boulders above the water that you can use to carefully work your way across. Otherwise, shoes are best left on

Location	Elevation	Distance from Previous Point	Cumulative Distance	UTM Coordinates
Silver Pass	10,750	—	0	11S 330017E 4148322N
Mott Lake junction	8980	3.7	3.7	11S 331341E 4145024N
Mono Creek junction	8350	1.4	5.1	11S 331029E 4143228N
Lake Edison junction	7900	1.4	6.5	11S 329758E 4142189N
Bear Ridge junction	9880	4.6	11.1	11S 330945E 4138822N
Bear Creek junction	8970	2.1	13.2	11S 332858E 4137219N
Hilgard Fork junction	9320	2.0	15.2	11S 333898E 4134673N
Bear Lakes junction	9570	1.2	16.4	11S 334661E 4132955N
Three Island Lake junction	10,015	1.1	17.5	11S 334429E 4131706N
Rose Lake junction	10,035	0.3	17.8	11S 334195E 4131442N
Marie Lake outlet	10,540	1.6	19.4	11S 334218E 4129774N
Selden Pass	10,890	0.9	20.3	11S 334070E 4128460N

SEE MAP 8

for this crossing. More switchbacks bring you to a crossing of the North Fork of Mono Creek, another very dangerous ford in early season, as the creekbed is rocky and the water turbulent, making footing difficult. (Having to make two such wretched crossings, one right after the other seems very unfair.) Immediately after the crossing you reach the junction with the trail to Mott Lake [8980' – 3.7/3.7] and a small campsite.

Just beyond the junction, you enter lush Pocket Meadow, filled with tall, yellow, sunflower-like flowers, orange sneezeweed. Soon, dry, rocky switchbacks resume. The presence of quaking aspens indicates areas subjected to disturbance, usually from avalanches. They are the first tree species to re-grow following such disturbance, and they often even continue to grow after being flattened by recurring avalanches. The bright blue, tubular flowers of showy penstemon greet you throughout the seemingly endless descent. At times, the grade lessens and you re-enter sections of mixed conifer forest and cross open slabs dotted with western junipers. After the junction with the Mono Pass Trail [8350' – 1.4/5.1], you turn westward to travel alongside Mono Creek. You continue descending, but the grade slowly eases, and you pass the first campsite in several miles. The forest now consists of towering Jeffrey pines, occasional western junipers, and stands of white fir. Shortly, you ford the North Fork of Mono Creek one last time. Once again, the water flow may be high and difficult, but at least here the river bottom is flat, broad, and covered with small pebbles (not boulders!). The next junction you reach, at Quail Meadows, is with the Lake Edison Trail [7900' – 1.4/6.5], which leads to the Lake Edison ferry landing and the Vermilion Valley Resort, a hospitable resupply stop for JMT and PCT travelers (see Appendix B). There is camping both near the trail junction beneath majestic Jeffrey pines, and a short distance off the JMT in Quail Meadows.

The JMT veers briefly east, to cross Mono Creek on a steel footbridge, and shortly begins the 2000-foot climb up Bear Ridge. There may be no water for the next 5 miles, up and over Bear Ridge, so it is advisable to fill your water bottles before beginning the ascent. Be sure to start the climb with enough daylight to reach the shoulder's far side. Fortunately, the trail is well graded and mostly under forest cover, making the interminable switchbacks more tolerable. About halfway up the climb, the trail sidles east toward a small, seasonal stream—a good place to dunk your head and cool off. At the base of the climb, western white pines, lodgepole pines, and a few western junipers dominate the tree cover, but with increasing elevation and changing slope, you will pass through many different conifer communities. Next, white

SEE MAP 8

firs dominate the forest, and then give way to a forest of western white pines, red firs, and mountain hemlocks. As the grade lessens, the forest is again a mix of lodgepole and western white pines, transitioning to pure lodgepole pine stands along the dry, flat sandy top of Bear Ridge. Ground cover has been variable but nearly always sparse, with creeping snowberry, rock cress, and alpine prickly currant as the most common species. The vegetation in the pure lodgepole pine stands is the least diverse, as these are the driest, sandiest soils. At the south end of Bear Ridge, you reach the junction with the Bear Ridge Trail, another alternative to reach Lake Thomas Edison [9880' – 4.6/11.1], and also the starting point for a detour to Volcanic Knob (see Appendix E).

The south side of Bear Ridge could not be more different from the landscape you just passed through: It is well watered, with many seeps covered by wildflowers and dense vegetation. The dry, sandy benches in between are dotted with western junipers. From many points, you have a beautiful vista north to Seven Gables. Among the many flowers dotting the wet landscape, two tall ones are ranger's buttons, with tall heads that bear many small, white balls of flowers on branching stalks, and arrow-leaved groundsel, with heads of small, straggly looking, yellow, daisy-like flowers, and large leaves shaped like acute triangles. Both are common species at nearly every stream crossing in the montane and subalpine zones. Several of the upper benches provide mediocre tent sites, but if you continue lower to an unmapped stream, you will encounter a large site beneath Jeffrey pines—a beautiful spot. Before long, the grade lessens, and you continue south across a wet slope, with small stream crossings and muddy sections, before reaching the Bear Creek Junction [8970' – 2.1/13.2]. This track leads to the Lake Thomas Edison area via the Bear Diversion Dam, providing the shortest access to the post office at Mono Hot Springs and, less directly, the Vermilion Valley Resort (see Appendix B).

Now in the beautiful canyon of rollicking Bear Creek, paralleling the creek on its east bank, the JMT begins a very gradual rise through lodgepole-pine-dominated forest, passing numerous campsites. Bear Creek, in stretches lined by granite slabs, contains enticing swimming holes when the water is low. In places, the lodgepole forest gives way to openings of dry sedge meadows. Common in these meadows are pretty faces, Leichtlin's mariposa lily, and Parish's yampah. Shortly, you reach the Hilgard Fork Trail junction, leading up to Lake Italy and then over Italy Pass on an unmaintained trail [9320' – 2.0/15.2]. You soon cross multi-stranded Hilgard Creek. You can cross the first two branches on logs, but you will likely need to wade the third during high

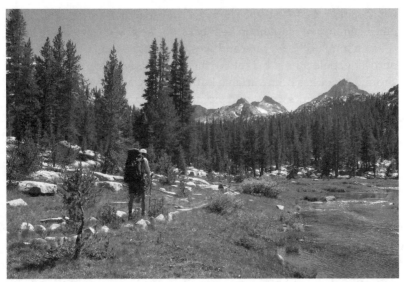

Walking through Rosemarie Meadow with Hooper Peak in the background

flow. There are campsites on either side of the crossings. Continuing through denser lodgepole forest, the JMT becomes faint in a marshy area; it trends slightly eastward. You next approach a trail that leads up the East Fork of Bear Creek [9570' – 1.2/16.4]. Just after the aforementioned trail junction, the JMT fords Bear Creek, which can be difficult in early season, especially since deep, swift water often combines with swarms of mosquitoes in this area. However, by late season, flow decreases and the abundant western blueberry bushes lining the banks of the stream may yield an appetizing snack.

Beyond the crossing, the grade increases to a moderate climb through dry lodgepole forest, leading to where the trail crosses the West Fork of Bear Creek, currently on a large log. There is a small and possibly muddy campsite east of the trail. Within 200 yards, you meet a trail that departs east for Three Island Lake and Lou Beverly Lake [10,015' – 1.1/17.5]. Before long, you enter charming Rosemarie Meadow, sporting good views of pyramid-shaped Mt. Hooper, a bit farther south. From the south end of the meadow, a trail climbs southwest to Rose Lake [10,035' – 0.3/17.8]. Open, wet subalpine to alpine meadows, like this one, are good places to spot either spotted sandpipers or water pipets, two birds that occur sporadically throughout the Sierra on high-elevation, wet, hummocky meadows. Lemmon's paintbrush, bog kalmia, dwarf bilberry, and primrose monkeyflower are all

SEE MAP 7

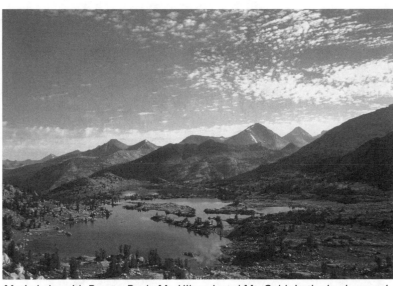

Marie Lake with Recess Peak, Mt. Hilgard, and Mt. Gabb in the background

common species here. Both Rose and Lou Beverly lakes provide good, secluded camping. Nearer the JMT, there are campsites in the slabs just above Rosemarie Meadow.

The trail now climbs steadily, passing scattered mountain hemlocks and whitebark pines, as it approaches Marie Lake. En route, you also pass a few large glacial erratics, notable because dark-colored rock fragments are embedded in an otherwise light-colored granite. This rock, originally from a small outcrop just east of Mt. Hooper, was transported downslope by a glacier. You are slowly climbing into the alpine, and much like on the north side of Silver Pass, the sandy soil is scattered with small plants that become noticeable only if you stare at your feet. Marie Lake fills a large, shallow basin trimmed and underlain by granite slabs, creating an oddly shaped lake dotted with islands. Several open campsites, often with open vistas northward, can be found on sandy patches near the outlet [10,540′ – 1.6/19.4]. You now skirt the lake's west shore and begin the final climb to Selden Pass. Be sure to turn and look northward, as the views of Marie Lake, with the peaks crowning the Mono Recesses in the background, are more open before you reach the summit. You will undoubtedly take another breather atop the pass, an almost quaint gap between granite walls and boulders [10,890′ – 0.9/20.3].

SEE MAP 7

SECTION 7.

Selden Pass to Muir Pass—South Fork of the San Joaquin River

Your final section within the San Joaquin drainage begins with a long downhill and ends with an even longer climb. It also marks a transition within your journey, as you pass the halfway point and then enter the ever-higher lake basins of the southern Sierra. As you begin your descent down rocky switchbacks, hunt for two related species, granite gilia and spreading phlox. Both have woody bases, needle-like leaves, and white, five-petal, somewhat tubular flowers. Granite gilia is taller and spinier, with petals whose bases form a tight cone, while the petal tips are more open. In contrast, spreading phlox crawls along the ground and has petals whose ends stick out at right angles. Descending both sandy, dry slopes and wetter ones, along seeps or small patches of meadow, you shortly pass little Heart Lake's east shore and cross its

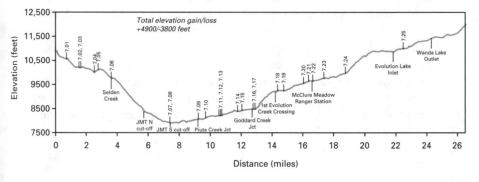

SEE MAP 7

outlet, Sallie Keyes Creek, twice. A small party will find a campsite near Heart Lake's outlet, exposed, but with open views. The JMT continues downward and shortly arrives at the upper Sallie Keyes Lake. The trail crosses Sallie Keyes Creek between the two lakes and follows the west shore of the lower lake. Along this stretch, there are many large campsites beneath lodgepole cover. A row of especially impressive lodgepole pines lines the bank of the lake; they are uncrowded and artistic, as if each were intentionally placed. At the outlet of the lower lake, you will cross Sallie Keyes Creek one final time on a logjam. In case of an emergency, there is sometimes a ranger staying at the snow survey cabin 0.4 mile south of the lakes, located on the east side of the trail.

Below Sallie Keyes Lakes, the JMT curves southeast through a meadow and then into open lodgepole forest. A short distance onward, and just after a more open knob, are a couple nice campsites. Water from a fork of Senger Creek is just a few more steps down the trail. You cross the creek and proceed through a very marshy meadow. More switchbacks, including a section passing large chinquapin-covered boulders, bring you to Senger Creek [9740' – 3.6/3.6]. Note that there are "no camping" postings for some areas on either side of the crossing;

Location	Elevation	Distance from Previous Point	Cumulative Distance	UTM Coordinates
Selden Pass	10,890	—	0	11S 334070E 4128460N
Senger Creek crossing	9740	3.6	3.6	11S 334734E 4124423N
JMT northern cutoff	8400	2.1	5.7	11S 334054E 4123186N
JMT southern cutoff	7880	1.7	7.4	11S 334959E 4121342N
Piute Creek junction	8050	1.8	9.2	11S 337415E 4121216N
Goddard Creek junction	8480	3.5	12.7	11S 340782E 4117608N
Wade across Evolution Creek	9200	1.5	14.2	11S 341941E 4117861N
McClure Meadow ranger station	9640	2.4	16.6	11S 345384E 4116969N
Evolution Lake inlet	10,852	5.2	21.8	11S 349861E 4113857N
Wanda Lake outlet	11,420	2.5	24.3	11S 349266E 4110347N
Muir Pass	11,980	2.2	26.5	11S 351636E 4108416N

SEE MAP 7

these signs are either for restoration or because the sites are too close to water, but legal campsites exist as well.

You now begin a long, dry drop into the river canyon far below. The grade is continuous, with no benches for camping. The open slope is mostly covered by large manzanita bushes and whitethorn, although a variety of other shrubs and herbs occasionally appear. Fox sparrows enjoy this vegetation and may be seen hopping in and out of the bushes. These brown, slightly streaked sparrows are a bit larger than others that you may be familiar with. Likely longing for shade, you slowly re-enter tree cover, mostly Jeffrey pines with scattered western junipers, and then reach a lateral to Florence Lake, the so-called "northern JMT cutoff" [8400' – 2.1/5.7]. It is thus known because this is the cutoff that southward walking JMT hikers take to reach either the Muir Trail Ranch, a food drop depot, or Florence Lake (see Appendix B for further route description). The hot pool at Blayney Hot Springs is also accessed by this trail, but crossing the San Joaquin to reach the hot springs can be dangerous, or impossible, during high flow. The JMT continues its traversing descent, still mostly through open Jeffrey pine forest, to reach the main branch of the Florence Lake Trail, or the "southern JMT cutoff" [7880' – 1.7/7.4]. If you have left the trail to pick up a food cache, and you do not too much mind missing a short stretch of the JMT, this is the junction where you will continue your southward journey on the JMT.

The JMT shortly diverges from the river, crossing over open, rocky, dry knobs of metamorphic rock with sedge meadows and scattered western junipers and Jeffrey pines. This open, flat valley of dark-colored rock is markedly different from anything you have seen to the north, or anything you will see to the south. Take your time to enjoy the majestic trees. Northern flickers, a species of woodpecker that feeds mostly on the ground, can be common at these elevations. They are easily identified by their red-orange underwings, visible in flight. Shortly, you reach a junction with the Piute Pass Trail, which goes north through Humphreys Basin and over Piute Pass to North Lake [8050' – 1.8/9.2]. As you cross turbulent Piute Creek on a steel footbridge, you leave behind John Muir Wilderness and enter Kings Canyon National Park. Nearby is a large, Jeffrey pine-shaded flat with numerous well-used and welcome campsites separated by chaparral thickets.

Leaving Piute Creek behind, the JMT begins a gradual traverse across the dry, sunny southwest canyon wall. Often far below the trail, the green waters of the South Fork of the San Joaquin River roll and tumble over ledges of dark, metamorphic rock. A Townsend's solitaire may be perched atop one of the western junipers, flying above the stream in search of insects. This brown bird is identified by the yellow-beige pattern visible on its wings when it flies and by its melodious song. Swarms of violet-green swallows also dive playfully above the water. By midseason, rufous hummingbirds are likely sucking nectar from the abundant flowers. At night, bats emerge, likely from crevices in the steep metamorphic wall to the west, to feed on insects. As you approach Aspen Meadow, you leave the open slopes behind. Moreover, the "meadow" is now a forest, a mixture of quaking aspen, lodgepole pine, white fir, and the occasional western juniper. There are several campsites during this forested stretch. You continue upstream, again in the open, taking in the impressive canyon walls and the turbulent waters. Common species on this dry slope include western eupatorium, a late-blooming species with a collection of light lavender heads, and many I have previously described, including granite gilia, scarlet penstemon, and small-leaved cream bush.

Shortly thereafter, you cross the river on a footbridge, pass a use trail to some campsites just northwest of the bridge, and continue upstream, now in lodgepole forest. The trail curves south, passing through drier and then wetter stretches of lodgepole forest as you head upstream. Alongside a small creek grow the bright orange Kelley's tiger lilies, sporting six reflexed petals. After an easy but possibly shoes-off creek crossing, you reach a junction where the Goddard Canyon/Hell For Sure Pass Trail continue south up the river, while the JMT turns east, crossing the South Fork of the San Joaquin on a log footbridge [8480' – 3.5/12.7].

Just over the bridge, the JMT hooks briefly north past some campsites before tackling east-trending switchbacks that take you up the canyon's steep east wall into one of the Sierra's most exquisite regions, hanging Evolution Valley. Take a breather as you climb, enjoy the panoramic vista, and especially look across to the west canyon wall. Note the streams and waterfalls flowing down deeply incised and nearly straight fractures in the metamorphic rock; granite rarely forms such straight, narrow channels down a cliff face. As the slope eases, the bedrock you are walking on again becomes granite, and Evolution Creek, to your north, changes character. Suddenly, you are walking alongside foaming cascades and deep, rounded holes, quite different from the steep-walled gorges a few miles back. The JMT presently leads to a creek crossing [9200' – 1.5/14.2]. Except under very high water, please cross here, as requested by the ranger-posted signs. This is the original

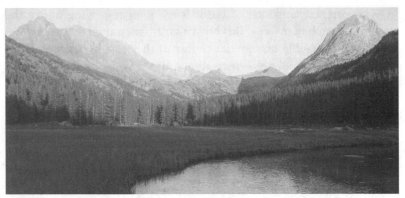

McClure Meadow with alpenglow on Mt. Mendel and the Hermit

crossing, which fell out of favor when a hole formed around a large rock in the channel.

As you continue upstream, around the northern edge of Evolution Meadow, you will pass several campsites occupying open areas beneath lodgepole cover. Along the trail, the forest floor is dry, except in areas with small seeps. In such areas, the swamp onion, with a tall stalk, purple flowers, and a pungent onion smell, is a common plant. Soon you reach McClure Meadow. A summer ranger is stationed on the slopes just north of the meadow, but the path to the cabin is easily missed if you are walking east [9640' – 2.4/16.6]. The campsites fringing McClure Meadow are justifiably popular for the views they offer—to the west lies a steep monolith, the Hermit, while along the eastern skyline are the first of the Evolution Basin peaks—Mt. Mendel, Mt. Darwin, Mt. Spencer, and Mt. Huxley. Continuing your gradual ascent and crossing several tributaries, you reach Colby Meadow and more campsites. Your route is still largely within dry lodgepole forest, with occasional excursions to the edge of meadows or onto granite slabs. Before long, you ford the multi-branched stream that drains Darwin Canyon; this is not difficult, but it is potentially cumbersome. Pass a small campsite on an open slab, and begin the climb to Evolution Basin. For the next 10 miles, there are few camping options, so if it is getting late in the day, consider stopping below this climb, and give yourself a full day to enjoy Evolution Basin.

If you look at the elevation profile for this section (on page 100) you will note that the distance from the low point, at the southern JMT cutoff, to the top of Muir Pass is divided into approximately three sections. First is the long, gradual climb up the South Fork of the San Joaquin, truncated by the abrupt climb as your leave Goddard Canyon for the hanging Evolution Valley. The many miles up Evolution Valley are again gentle, but you now leave Evolution Valley and climb steeply up into another hanging valley, in which Evolution Basin and its famous lakes are found. A hanging valley forms when the glacier in the side valley cannot erode its valley floor as quickly as does the glacier in the main valley, creating a steep drop-off. At the first step, Goddard Canyon was eroded more quickly than Evolution Valley, and at the second, the drainage to the McGee Lakes was more eroded than Evolution Basin.

Just at the top of the last switchback is the unsigned junction with a use trail to spectacular Darwin Bench, well worth a detour to camp or eat lunch, or, alternatively, up over Lamarck Col, a popular cross-country route. As the gradient lessens, the forest thins, the views open up, and you find yourself walking on sand patches between granite slabs and rocky outcrops. Such habitat is ideal for the white-tailed ptarmigan, an introduced species whose population remarkably stabilized at relatively low numbers.

Within a short distance, you leave the last stunted trees behind, reach the outlet of Evolution Lake, find a few small campsites north of the lake's outlet, and look forward to your 5-mile tromp through undeniably spectacular Evolution Basin. Make sure you have many hours to wander upward and to sit and stare. This basin is also steeped in JMT history: In July 1895, Theodore Solomons, the visionary of the JMT, named the first six peaks of the Evolution Range after the most prominent figures in the new field of evolutionary biology: Darwin, Fiske, Haeckel, Huxley, Spencer, and Wallace, along with Evolution Lake. Although Solomons had first alighted on the idea of the JMT a decade earlier, it was on trips in 1895 and 1896 that he fleshed out his idea, in part while soaking up the landscape of Evolution Basin. During these summers, he traveled along the current JMT route as far as Muir Pass, but his parties then descended to the Middle Fork of the Kings by other routes. Their goal was to find a route between Yosemite and the South Fork of the Kings that stayed close to the crest and was passable by stock. Both years, then unnamed Muir Pass was buried beneath an enormous snow bank, and they searched farther west for alternatives. Finally, in 1907, a US Geological Survey party crossed Muir Pass, and the following year, Joseph N. Le Conte used the pass as he continued scouting a route for the eventual JMT. You skirt around the eastern shore of Evolution Lake, on a route constructed in the early 1990s to avoid the lake's sensitive shoreline. You are passing by the massive wall of scalloped ridges and gullies descending from Mt. Mendel, a later-named addition to the Evolution Peaks. Shortly, you reach Evolution Lake's inlet, crossed on a series of large granite blocks [10,852′

SEE MAP 6

– 5.2/21.8]. You continue up a gentle slope, passing sandy stretches dotted with small alpine plants, meadows dotted with a more colorful selection of flowers, and to the east, a series of small lakes. The sandy flats often contain Muir's ivesia, one of the few plants to bear the name of this famous naturalist. These are small yellow flowers on long stalks with dense stalks of minute, fuzzy leaves that resemble a mouse's tail. In these same stretches, you may see the alpine paintbrush, not as dazzling and bright as the other species, but still elegantly colored. Growing just a few inches off the ground, the characteristic tubular flowers range from green to white to light pink, and the upper leaves sport a dainty white or pink edge. Meanwhile, Lemmon's paintbrush, with the magenta flowers, grows in the wetter meadows you pass. This is also the habitat of gray-crowned rosy finches, delightful little birds. They are common at high elevations, traveling in small groups and feeding on the insects that emerge from the alpine tarns or scavenging them from snow banks.

Near the outlet of stunning Sapphire Lake, the trail begins to climb up the west side of the valley. If you were to leave the JMT here and head around the eastern shore of Sapphire Lake, you would find a few small campsites among the whitebark pines at the southern end of the lake. This is also the point to leave the trail if you wish to climb Mt. Spencer, which is markedly steep as you approached from the north, but has an easy ascent from the southwest (see Appendix E). The grade eases again as you approach a pair of unnamed lakes. As you make this climb, stop and admire the many glacial features that surround you. During the last ice age, Evolution Basin was scoured clean, and the abundant glacial erratics scattered across the landscape attest to the glaciers' presence. Since then, little soil formation has occurred, and the smooth granite slabs still dominate the landscape. Meanwhile, the upper sections of the highest peaks, Mt. Darwin and Mt. Mendel, were untouched by glaciers. Their summit regions are broad plateaus, the remnants of a gentle Sierra landscape that existed before a combination of uplift and river erosion, followed by glacial activity, created today's landforms. Take note of the chutes and ribs that decorate their western faces—these are avalanche chutes, whose exact locations are determined by the location of joints within the granite. The rock in the joints is more easily fractured and displaced by freeze-thaw activity, and the loose rock is then carried downslope by the snow. In many places in the Sierra, these avalanches not only remove rock, but also polish the chutes. As you continue down the trail, note that these giant slides are often truncated some distance above today's valley floor, at the boundary between "steep chute" and "nearly vertical wall," marking the height to which the valley was once filled with ice.

SEE MAPS 5-6

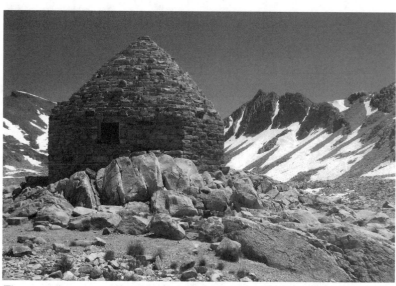

The stone hut atop Muir Pass with the Black Giant peering out to the left

You now cross the multi-branched outlet [11,420′ − 2.5/24.3] of Wanda Lake and soon reach the large lake, named for one of John Muir's daughters. To the southwest rises the massive, dark pyramid of Mt. Goddard, the tallest of the peaks in the Ionian Basin, hidden to the south. This black rock comprises the Goddard Terrane, one of the largest masses of metamorphic rock in the Sierra. The action of plate tectonics smashed material into the continent between 150 million and 250 million years ago, leading to large volcanic eruptions. The subsequent tectonic action that created the Sierra Nevada's granite caused the volcanic rock to be metamorphosed, creating the dark rock you will see to the south of the trail for the next many miles. The JMT skirts the metamorphic rock, but you can obtain a good view of the Ionian Basin with its crystal clear aqua lakes by climbing Mt. Solomons, from Muir Pass. You can get a good view of the rock itself by ascending the Black Giant, a bit further southeast (see Appendix E).

Your trail follows Wanda's grassy east shore before climbing gradually past Lake McDermand and up to Muir Pass [11,980′ − 2.2/26.5], where there is a stone hut intended to provide emergency shelter from storms. Camping in the area is prohibited because of human-waste problems. A marmot is always on guard at the hut; keep your eyes on your food at all times!

SEE MAPS 5–6

SECTION 8.

Muir Pass to Mather Pass— Middle Fork of the Kings River

A s you cross Muir Pass, you are entering the Kings River drainage. With the exception of the 5 miles in the Rush Creek drainage, all the land you have traversed thus far drains into the San Francisco Bay. From here south, water reaches the ocean only in wet years—mind-boggling when you consider the vast quantities of snow that bury this country each winter! The water from the Kings and Kern drainages once flowed into Tulare Lake in the southern San Joaquin Valley, a vast wetland, but today *all* of the water is diverted for irrigation, and the Tulare lakebed is mostly agricultural land.

Vindicating Solomons for overlooking the relatively straightfor-ward Muir Pass, snow does often linger on the east side of Muir Pass well into the summer, and you descend toward Helen Lake on either rocky-sandy switchbacks or across a well-trodden path in the snow. To

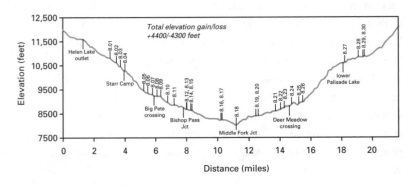

 SEE MAP 5

the southeast lies the Black Giant, the northern end of the metamorphic Black Divide and an easy peak with an excellent vista if you have half a day to spare (see Appendix E). As you encircle Helen Lake, named for John Muir's other daughter, enjoy its brilliant blue waters and the surrounding colorful glaciated slabs. The trail passes near the contact between metamorphic and granitic rocks, and shortly crosses Helen Lake's outlet [11,615' – 1.3/1.3]. You follow the infant Middle Fork of the Kings River down an enticing little gorge, paved with dark rock. For stretches, the creek flows over the trail, but it is too small to impede your progress. Flowers appreciate the abundant moisture and color the base of steep walls. One species is the mountain monkeyflower, similar in shape to the primrose monkeyflower but much larger and growing in seeps, rather than meadows. Shortly, you reach a small, unnamed lake and follow the trail across the inlet stream, where the water spreads out into a meadow filled with dense patches of mountaineer shooting stars interspersed with cobble-paved waterways.

You continue downstream, passing knobs of metamorphic rock, cross back into granite, and shortly view your first stunted whitebark pine since Evolution Lake. Take note that granitic knobs are much more likely than metamorphic ones to contain small, flat, sandy patches that suffice as small campsites. Just above the 10,800-foot mark, you ford another series of inlet streams and encircle another unnamed lake. Good

Location	Elevation	Distance from Previous Point	Cumulative Distance	UTM Coordinates
Muir Pass	11,980	—	0	11S 351636E 4108416N
Helen Lake outlet	11,615	1.3	1.3	11S 352659E 4109140N
Starr Camp	10,480	2.3	3.6	11S 354585E 4108611N
Big Pete Meadow creek crossing	9245	2.3	5.9	11S 357303E 4108387N
Bishop Pass junction	8720	1.9	7.8	11S 358398E 4106234N
Middle Fork junction	8070	3.4	11.2	11S 359647E 4101681N
Deer Meadow creek crossing	8830	3.4	14.6	11S 364338E 4101912N
Lower Palisade Lake outlet	10,615	3.5	18.1	11S 367705E 4102392N
Mather Pass	12,100	3.6	21.7	11S 370227E 4099161N

SEE MAP 5

campsites with stunning views lie among the stunted trees on the knob to the east of its outlet. The JMT continues downward, switchbacking down a steeper slope, crossing the creek several times. Trickles of water abound, and the vegetation is lush, with mountaineer shooting stars, Labrador tea, red heather, and Sierra arnica all making appearances. Clark's nutcrackers will be hopping among the treetops. Gaze up at the looming east face of the Black Giant and note how the peak's character changes at the contact between metamorphic and granitic rocks. A few large campsites present themselves under open stands of tall lodgepole pines. You pass a large, marshy meadow and then a flat of young lodgepole pines, long-ago named Starrs Camp. If you leave the trail here, you find abundant camping opportunities in the direction of the creek, positioned at the top of the steep drop into Le Conte Canyon [10,480' – 2.3/3.6].

The stream now plunges downward and the trail switchbacks a bit more gradually down the north canyon wall through patchy forest. In wet sections, you will see large ferns and fireweed, which have clusters of quite large, four-petal pink flowers on very tall stalks. Drier sections are dominated by shrubs, including manzanita and chinquapin. To navigate through one section, the trail had to be blasted out of the canyon's sheer granite wall, and when you read Joseph N. Le Conte's account of crisscrossing the valley multiple times to navigate around the cliffs, you'll be glad for the work of the dynamite. The trail becomes ever rockier underfoot, as you pound down increasingly dry slopes toward the valley bottom. Suddenly, the trail intersects the stream course, you re-enter the forest, and there again campsites. Although there are stands of mountain hemlocks on steep, north-facing slopes, the river-bottom forest is dominated by lodgepole pines. You walk along the refreshingly soft trail through the forest, shortly crossing, on logs, the multi-branched side stream that intersects the trail just before Big Pete Meadow [9245' – 2.3/5.9]. Just after the crossing, you pass several small campsites and, farther along, a spur trail that leads to larger campsites along the main stream. For a short stretch, you emerge from the lodgepole forest onto a sandy slope with western junipers and phenomenal views westward to the steep face of Languille Peak. There is one small campsite here. You next come to Little Pete Meadow, which is, contrary to its name, large. A stream meanders through here. Oxbow lakes, which formed when the stream changed its course, are visible as well. To the edge are dense stands of corn lilies: Early in the season, these look like ears of corn, but by summer they are taller and straggly. A few of these plants will have many-branched heads of white flowers, but most senesce without flowering. There are a few campsites along the meadow's perimeter. Soon thereafter, the JMT reaches the spur trail to the Le Conte Canyon ranger station and, just thereafter, a junction with the Bishop Pass Trail [8720' – 1.9/7.8], leading up into Dusy Basin and over Bishop Pass, the easiest route to the town of Bishop.

Along the stretch of trail from here to the confluence of the Middle Fork of the Kings River and Palisade Creek, there are few campsites that are 100 feet from the trail and/or water. Remember that the Kings Canyon regulations do allow you to camp in established campsites that are 25 feet from trail/water. You immediately pass a few campsites and then cross the turbulent Dusy Branch on a footbridge. For stretches you are walking through dry, predominately lodgepole forest; for others, you head across dry, open slopes, often where avalanches or rockslides prevent a conifer forest from establishing. Slopes covered by downslope-oriented tree trunks and vegetated by scrubby aspens are indicative of avalanche activity. In these open sections, note a mixture of two different manzanitas. One, pinemat manzanita creeps along the ground, often under scattered tree cover, while the other, greenleaf manzanita, grows as a taller bush and has sticky glands on its leaf stalks. Both have scaly red bark, characteristic of all manzanita species. A few miles downstream, the trail passes Grouse Meadow, a long, skinny meadow with outstanding views of Le Conte Canyon and with one of the largest blueberry patches in the Sierra. You will find several campsites along its length. You continue downstream to the Middle Fork Trail junction [8070' – 3.4/11.2], your lowest point until after the summit of Mt. Whitney. Several campsites are present here beneath tall Jeffrey pines. In the past, you could cross Palisade Creek on a bridge, but a flood has washed out all but the foundation, visible a short distance upstream, and the trail down the Middle Fork of the Kings is now difficult to access if water is high. To continue your history lesson: Until the switchbacks up the Golden Staircase, 3 miles ahead, were completed, hikers continued descending the Middle Fork of the Kings and then ascended Cartridge Creek, some miles west.

The JMT now turns eastward and, paralleling Palisade Creek, begins its long climb to Mather Pass. The next many miles have fewer campsites than in the past: Some sections are overgrown with aspen scrub, and much of the next 3 miles was affected by the 2002 lightning-started Palisade Fire. The trail is often indistinct as its passes through meadows, and there are downed trees from winter, making travel a bit slow in places. As the vegetation changes during the next many years, the location of campsites will change, but the best opportunities are undisturbed stands of trees near the river or sandy shelves under Jeffrey pines to the north of the trail. Although there is now less forest cover, the herbaceous cover is lush and diverse. Just before Deer Meadow, you re-enter undisturbed lodgepole forest and cross the stream draining Palisade Basin high above [8830′ – 3.4/14.6]. Heading south from the trail, you find a couple of shaded campsites in Deer Meadow, a lodgepole forest. An often-marshy section of trail then crosses many forks of Glacier Creek, draining another basin at the foot of the 14,000-foot northern Palisade Peaks, and enters another section of dense lodgepole forest with several camping opportunities.

You shortly exit forest cover and begin an exposed 1500-foot climb up switchbacks known as the Golden Staircase. Impressively built walls form the foundation for the switchbacks that make for a steep climb up a much steeper headwall. Completed in 1938, this was the last section of the JMT to be constructed, and the only section of the route that Le Conte was unable to navigate with stock on his 1908 expedition. For stretches, the trail is dry and rocky, while elsewhere small seeps provide water and host a different community of plants. The drier sections are dominated by the ever more familiar wavy-leaved paintbrush, scarlet penstemon, pennyroyal, and western eupatorium. The wetter sections boast orange sneezeweed, swamp onion, Kelley's tiger lily, and great red paintbrush. Two other species in the wetter sites are the Sierra rein orchid, bearing very small, white, orchid-shaped flowers on leafy stalks, and alpine goldenrod, with short, yellow, ray petals that look dwarfed relative to the size of the orange-yellow disc. As you climb higher, look along rocky walls for a pink-flowered shrub whose stems emerge from cracks and branches literally hug the rock: cliff bush. But also take breaks from staring at your feet, and look south to tumbling Palisade Creek, taking the direct route to Deer Meadow, and west to Devils Crags, the dark, jagged mass of pinnacles at the southern end of the Black Divide. The grade eases in a pretty alpine meadow just below lower Palisade Lake, where you have your first awe-inspiring view of the 14,000-foot Palisades. After fording a couple of tributaries, you reach the west end of the lower Palisade Lake [10,615′ – 3.5/18.1], where, on slabs to the north of the trail, there is one large campsite. It is sandy and barren, but what views!

The trail bends southeastward, as it skirts the northeastern shores of the Palisade Lakes. You will see the steep granite walls to the south, the sharp-toothed Middle Palisade group to the north, and Mather Pass to the east. You ford an occasional stream, some of which may require a brief wade in early season, and while traversing high above the

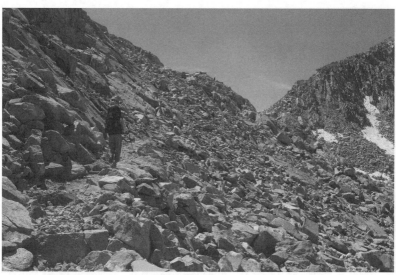

Hiking past giant talus blocks on the ascent to Mather Pass

upper Palisade Lake, pass several view-rich campsites on small shelves amongst stunted whitebark pines. Once past the lakes, the trail turns south, traverses small meadows and soon begins the final ascent to the pass: switchbacks through amazingly barren talus. One species that frequently grows along the base of talus blocks is the bright pink Sierra primrose. It is a southern Sierra species that is quite rare farther north in the Sierra. In cracks in slabs emerge clumps of stalks topped by tufts of yellow flowers. These are club-moss ivesia, which are widespread and become one of the dominant species at the highest elevations, always emerging from such cracks. Finally, you reach Mather Pass, named for Stephen Mather, the first head of the National Park Service, and enjoy a much-deserved break on the summit [12,100′ – 3.6/21.7]. Looking back northward, you see the full length of the North and Middle Palisade peaks: Within view are six points that extend above the 14,000-foot mark.

SEE MAP 4

SECTION 9.

Mather Pass to Pinchot Pass— South Fork of the Kings River

The view south from Mather Pass is equally fantastic: To the east is Split Mountain, the southernmost of the Palisade-area fourteeners. If you wish to take a layover day in the vicinity, it is a straightforward, if long, climb (see Appendix E). Due south, where you are headed next, is another of the JMT's spectacular alpine basins, lake-dotted Upper Basin, the headwaters of the South Fork of the Kings River. You descend moderately, curving first east, and then resuming a southern bearing, as you enter Upper Basin. Although no established campsites are visible from the trail, you can easily wander toward any of the tarns and may pitch your tent on flat, sandy, unvegetated patches. The scale of these tarns is so different from Evolution Basin's deep, giant lakes, but they are equally enticing. You can so easily sit along their banks, sometimes on nearly bare sand, other times on polished slabs, and stare at the collection of insects and perhaps small tadpoles racing about.

You continue downslope, crossing a few small tributaries en route. The gentle grade makes for easy going—all the better to appreciate the

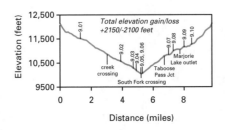

SEE MAP 4

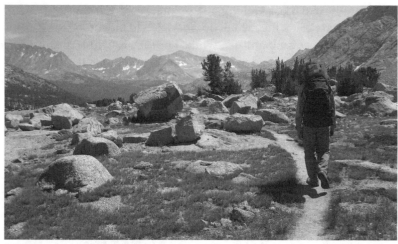

Hiking through Upper Basin with views south to Pinchot Pass

landscape. To the west are steep, glaciated granite peaks, and to the east, craggy, colorful metamorphic ones. For the next many miles, you are close to the contact between the older metamorphic rocks and the younger granitic ones. Like the rocks comprising the Goddard Terrane around Muir Pass, the precursors to these metamorphic rocks formed in place: seafloor-deposited sediments that were later compressed and twisted. This material, termed roof pendants, once overlay the granite through much of the Sierra, but it was eroded across much of the range as the granite core was uplifted, first about 50 million years ago, and

Location	Elevation	Distance from Previous Point	Cumulative Distance	UTM Coordinates
Mather Pass	12,100	—	0	11S 370227E 4099161N
South Fork Kings crossing at base of Upper Basin	10,860	3.0	3.0	11S 370783E 4095789N
Main South Fork Kings crossing	10,040	2.2	5.2	11S 371517E 4092357N
Taboose Pass junction	10,780	1.5	6.7	11S 371999E 4091458N
Crossing below Lake Marjorie	11,055	1.0	7.7	11S 372474E 4090150N
Pinchot Pass	12,130	2.1	9.8	11S 374301E 4088514N

SEE MAP 4

more rapidly in the last 3 million to 5 million years. Cardinal Mountain, a massive red peak with a white tip, sticks out to the southeast: The red material was once sand and silt, while the white is marble, the remains of ocean critters deposited in a shallow reef environment.

Forest cover increases as you descend and again ford the river near some campsites [10,860' – 3.0/3.0]. Over the next mile, snooping eastward, in the direction of the river, can yield additional camping opportunities. Soon you are in a lodgepole forest, many sections with enough moisture for denser than usual understory vegetation. Near some good campsites, a rock cairn marks where an old trail, whose route you can still follow, climbs to Taboose Pass. Farther downstream, another old (although not quite vanished) trail descends the South Fork of the Kings, before climbing over Cartridge Pass, through Lakes Basin, and down Cartridge Creek, the route of the JMT used temporarily while the trail up the Golden Staircase and Mather Pass were being built. Soon you reach the main crossing of the South Fork of the Kings [10,040' – 2.2/5.2], which can be quite difficult: In early season, you will want to wade across where the river splits around an islet downstream, and later in the season, you can hop across rocks a bit upstream. Some campsites near this crossing may be closed for restoration, but options abound.

Shortly after the first crossing, you ford a tributary and then begin a dry, switchbacking ascent southward through open lodgepole forest. One common plant on dry, south-facing slopes is Nuttall's sandwort, a straggly, mat-like plant with small, star-shaped, white flowers and needle-shaped leaves. The steep climb ends as you reach a junction with the Taboose Pass Trail [10,780' – 1.5/6.7]. Within minutes, you step across a small trickle and then ford the creek draining from Pinchot Pass. Just beyond is the signed junction with the Bench Lake Trail. If you have extra energy to walk another 2 miles, Bench Lake, perched high above the South Fork of the Kings River, has beautiful campsites along its northeastern shore, sporting justifiably famous sunrise reflections of Arrow Peak.

A short distance south along the JMT is the Bench Lake ranger station, located on the northeast shore of the first lake you reach; note that this ranger station is not always staffed. As you walk, be sure to stop and look north to Mather Pass: The impressively steep peak just north of the South Fork of the Kings is Mt. Ruskin. Small campsites exist on sandy, slightly forested knobs to the side of most of the next several tarns you pass. Their outlets are all easily crossed, mostly on large blocks of rock. The final crossing is just downstream of the last tarn before Lake Marjorie [11,055' – 1.0/7.7]. Between this crossing

SEE MAP 4

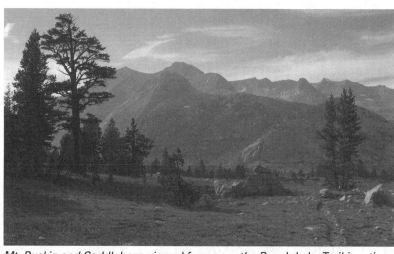

Mt. Ruskin and Saddlehorn viewed from near the Bench Lake Trail junction

and Lake Marjorie, you can find small tent sites tucked away in sandy patches beneath the stunted whitebark pines, including some near Lake Marjorie's outlet.

The JMT traces Lake Marjorie's eastern shore and ascends past the last krumholz. Your final miles to Pinchot Pass are very different from those ascending Mather Pass. You are in orange metamorphic rock, which decomposes to form a richer soil, and water is more abundant. Therefore, instead of switchbacking through endless talus, you cross little meadows and creeks, covered by an enormous diversity of plants. A few sandy patches even provide campsites not far below the pass. On moist slopes, you will pass shrubs covered with bright yellow flowers, each of whose five petals approximate the shape of a rose petal; it is bush cinquefoil, a member of the rose family. Wet meadows are covered with primrose monkeyflower, Sierra penstemon, little elephant's head, and alpine aster, a purple daisy, always with a single head, whose petals are incurved where they attach to the central disc. Small, sandy flats are covered by masses of short, red, straggly stems, the remains of early-blooming bud saxifrage. The last climb to the pass is then dominated by talus species, including many requiring wet conditions, such as the delightful Eschscholtz's buttercup, always growing in the wettest patches and identified by its deeply lobed leaves. Of course, in contrast to steep-sided granite peaks, the much fractured metamorphic rock leads to peaks that are piles of lose scree. Soon you are on the summit of the pass, looking back one last time to Mather Pass and Upper Basin [12,130′ – 2.1/9.8].

SEE MAP 4

SECTION 10.

Pinchot Pass to Glen Pass—Woods Creek Fork of the Kings River

Looking south from Pinchot Pass, you take in the next magnificent alpine basin—once again meadows and little tarns, surrounded by red metamorphic mountains on most sides. This drainage, Woods Creek, is a tributary of the South Fork of the Kings River; their confluence is in Paradise Valley, approximately 4 miles downstream of where the JMT crosses Woods Creek. Down you go on tight switchbacks, then across flower-strewn alpine meadows, stepping across a streamlet here and there. Crater Mountain, to the west, has an amazing vista south to the King Spur if you have half a day to spare (see Appendix E). Once you are past the uppermost meadows, the JMT curves east to traverse above an enchanting series of ponds and lakes—if you don't have time for a break now, come back just to visit them someday. The

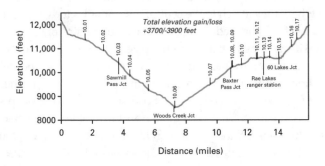

SEE MAP 4

trail has been rerouted and now stays high to avoid damaging the delicate meadow vegetation; you are instead traversing through short sections of talus and rocky outcrops, interspersed by long, sandy stretches. Only once down below 11,000 feet do you skirt the edge of a small lake, where there is camping on small knobs to the east of the trail. The trail continues downward, alternatively in sections of whitebark and lodgepole forest, across mostly metamorphic slabs and sandy patches, and through dry sedge meadows. The latter are often dotted with small, yellow flowers resembling dandelions: alpineflames. Elsewhere, you may have seen the superficially similar short-beaked agoseris, but this species lacks the central disc seen in the alpineflames, such that the multi-lengthed ray petals merge to a single point. You pass the signed junction to the trail northeast to Sawmill Pass [10,345' – 3.7/3.7]; a few exposed campsites lie on the bench just east of this junction, across the multistranded creek.

Descending more steeply now, the JMT drops into the sun-struck, southwest-trending canyon of Woods Creek, passing a good campsite near 9850 feet, just where the trail crosses a side creek and leaves forest cover. You next cross beneath a long talus field dotted with tall lupines, willows, scarlet penstemon, pennyroyal, and wavy-leaved paintbrush. One not-yet-mentioned species is Sierra angelica, sporting an enormous spherical head of miniature white flowers on a tall stalk. The trail now follows the creek's northern shore, often providing good views of the small stream gorge and at one point of some small cascades. On one small bench are the first foxtail pines that you have seen; this southern Sierra species will shortly become much more common in the subalpine

Location	Elevation	Distance from Previous Point	Cumulative Distance	UTM Coordinates
Pinchot Pass	12,130	—	0	11S 374301E 4088514N
Sawmill Pass junction	10,345	3.7	3.7	11S 375312E 4084783N
Woods Creek junction	8492	3.5	7.2	11S 371810E 4081629N
Baxter Pass junction	10,200	3.7	10.9	11S 374508E 4077248N
Rae Lakes ranger station	10,580	2.1	13.0	11S 375124E 4074637N
60 Lakes Basin junction	10,545	1.0	14.0	11S 374962E 4073715N
Glen Pass	11,940	1.9	15.9	11S 374134E 4072250N

SEE MAPS 3–4

zone. Farther along this same bench are a collection of campsites, mostly quite small. Shortly thereafter, you ford the White Fork tributary, possibly difficult early in the season. Around this elevation, you descend back into the realm of towering Jeffrey pines and, a bit later, western junipers as well. On the other side of the creek, you observe a well-delineated moraine, the piles of material pushed to the side by a glacier that once flowed down this canyon. The trail takes you ever deeper into the canyon, crossing several more tributaries. Although these will all be wades in early season, the crossings are flat, with good foot purchase on small- to medium-sized rocks. Stare at the now towering walls around you, Castle Domes to the north and the King Spur to the south, and the stream cascading down smooth slabs. You now descend the final manzanita-covered slope to the trail junction with the Woods Creek Trail [8492' – 3.5/7.2], which goes south down Woods Creek, past Paradise Valley, to Cedar Grove.

At the junction, you trend south and southeast on the overgrown north bank to cross roaring Woods Creek on an imposing, narrow, and very bouncy suspension bridge known as the "Golden Gate of the Sierra." It was completed in 1988 and is not subject to washouts like its predecessor. (One person at a time, please.) On the south bank, beneath Jeffrey pines, red firs, and a few lodgepole pines, is a large camping area and two bear boxes. South of the trail are additional campsites near a juniper-covered knob. Note that for the next many miles up to and through the Rae Lakes Basin, there are a few large campsites, but only marginal camping opportunities in between, so you can expect company each night. As you continue up the South Fork of Woods Creek, you pass through many vegetation communities: The first stretch is through open lodgepole forest, where a cobble-covered forest floor provides evidence of past flood events. Higher up, long sections cross dry, open knobs with small sedge meadows and slabs on which mountain-pride penstemon, mountain sagebrush, Nuttall's sandwort, and wavy-leaved paintbrush are usually common. About 1.5 miles upstream of the Woods Creek crossing, you ford a stream draining lakes on the northern tip of the King Spur; the water can be deep in early season. Another mile upstream, you pass a large, marshy meadow filled with wildflowers. By late season, three species of gentian will be blooming here: the stalkless, white-colored alpine gentian; Sierra gentian, with a single, narrow, tubular, purple flower on a 4-inch stalk; and the periwinkle-colored perennial swertia, with numerous flowers on an 8-inch stalk. By August, the alpine gentian and Sierra gentian are widespread meadow constituents. Several species of orchids, many with small,

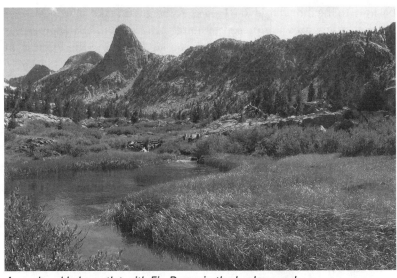

Arrowhead Lake outlet with Fin Dome in the background

white-green flowers, are also present here. Shortly thereafter, you re-intersect the main drainage and can find a small campsite downstream of the trail. As you continue upstream, the terrain becomes ever rockier and drier. Foxtail pines slowly replace the lodgepole pines, and by the time you emerge onto dark-colored granitic slabs, you are in a stark landscape of scattered foxtail pines. Their long, dangling branches often have needles only near the tip, where they encircle the stem like a bottlebrush. Where the slope lessens, you reach Dollar Lake and the junction with the Baxter Pass Trail [10,200' – 3.7/10.9].

This marks the beginning of the Rae Lakes Basin, a scenic and highly used area with a well-earned reputation for bad mosquitoes. Be sure to read the regulations that are posted at the junction. There are a few campsites near Dollar Lake and more a short distance upstream at Arrowhead Lake. Both are beautiful locations with excellent sunset and sunrise reflections of Fin Dome, the prominent, steep granite dome a bit upstream. Dollar Lake is more exposed, and you camp on open, sandy patches among granite slabs; Arrowhead Lake's campsites are under lodgepole forest near a bear box, and the lake is ringed by a large meadow and reeds. Above Arrowhead Lake, you continue climbing through lodgepole forest. Along your trek, you may have noted a burgundy-colored succulent, especially prominent in rocky seeps. This is rosy sedum, and it also occurs sporadically in this stretch of forest. As you approach Fin Dome, the grade eases and you reach the upper

SEE MAP 3

basin with the three large Rae Lakes. At the lowest lake, a bear box and large camping area are present among scattered whitebark pines. As you traipse up-canyon, you next pass a sign marking the location of the Rae Lakes ranger station, a short distance east of the trail [10,580′ − 2.1/13.0]. Your traverse along the east side of the lakes is lovely; you cross many little flower-filled seeps and look out across the lakes and westward to the steep peaks of the King Spur: Mt. Cotter and Mt. Clarence King. As you continue around the middle Rae Lake, the views to the south and east become enticing as well—colorful metamorphic rock, especially on the face of the Painted Lady at the head of the canyon, and the blocky outline of the Sierra Crest near Dragon Peak. Thanks to the marshy meadows, seeps, and many lakes, birds are also abundant in this basin: Yellow-rumped warblers, the all-yellow Wilson's warblers, and white-crowned sparrows are likely darting in an out of willows at the edge of meadows; Clark's nutcrackers will be congregating in whitebark pines. Near the south end of the middle Rae Lake, a sign points you toward the lake's shore, where there is a large camping area with bear boxes. You cross between the middle and upper Rae Lakes on a narrow isthmus (no camping allowed here) and, just after fording the connecting stream, you reach the junction to the Sixty Lakes Basin [10,545′ − 1.0/14.0]. Scattered campsites exist west and northwest of the junction. This exquisite subalpine basin is worth exploring if you have a few hours to spare, as the views of Mt. Clarence King are even more sublime, and the lakes are exquisite.

From this junction, you begin the switchbacking climb to Glen Pass. Keep your eyes open as you climb, as these next miles are where you are most likely to see Sierra Nevada bighorn sheep. You pass through sheep habitat several times on your journey, but the animals are both rare and difficult to spot—boulders with legs, in the words of one researcher. However, for the last several years, a herd of rams has often been spotted here atop rocky knobs or in talus. Your climb begins under scattered tree cover, with an understory often dominated by red mountain heather, but as you climb, you are increasingly switchbacking amongst slabs and an occasional creek. Knobs to the east of the trail provide small campsites with views down-canyon. The slope briefly flattens as you cross talus and slabs in a basin of austere mountain tarns. A few minute sandy patches may beckon to you as campsites, but, unfortunately, they are only visible once you are five minutes up the trail and above them. If you wish to detour to climb the Painted Lady, which offers an outstanding aerial view of the Rae Lakes, it is on this flat that you leave the trail (see Appendix E). The vegetation from

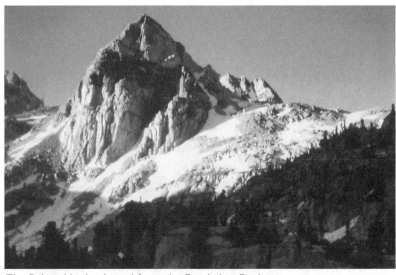

The Painted Lady viewed from the Rae Lakes Basin

here to the summit is remarkably sparse; a few sections sport dense patches of Sierra primrose, and cracks in outcrops are again filled with club-moss ivesia, with its tufts of small yellow flowers. Three other species might also engage your eye as your puff upwards: Mountain sorrel grows beneath shaded boulders and is identified by its rounded leaves and elongated stalks of either white flowers or red seeds; Sierra fleabane daisy, another common member of the fellfield community, has a dense head of up to 120 purple ray petals; granite (or Lemmon's) draba is a cushion plant that is ubiquitous under moist boulders. It is a type of mustard with small, four-petal, yellow flowers that cover the top of the cushion when in bloom. The higher you rise, the more often you should pause to enjoy the view northward: Great peaks dominate a barren, rocky, brown, lake-speckled world with precious little green of tree or meadow visible—and yet, having just passed through it, you know the area is rich with beautiful lakes and streams, trees, meadows, and wildflowers. The final few switchbacks often hold snow throughout the season, and then you finally stand atop windy, narrow Glen Pass [11,960' – 1.9/15.9].

SEE MAP 3

SECTION 11.

Glen Pass to
Forester Pass—Bubbs Creek Fork
of the Kings River

The southern side of Glen Pass drains into Bubbs Creek, another fork of the South Fork of the Kings; the two merge in Cedar Grove, approximately 18 trail miles to the west. Your view south from Glen Pass is mostly blocked by the steep-walled cirque into which you will descend. However, to the southwest, you can see the northern tip of the Great Western Divide: pyramid-shaped Mt. Brewer flanked by the unimpressive South Guard and notably steep North Guard. Switchbacks take you down a dry, loose, scree slope to a couple of pothole lakes and a seasonal alpine stream. As always, the ground becomes more vegetated as the grade lessens, in this case with red mountain heather and Sierra primroses growing among boulders. A few small tent sites are nestled among the whitebark pines on the southwest side of the first lake. You

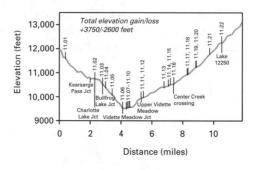

SEE MAP 3

descend more switchbacks to a second lake. As you pass it, look south-east at the steep-fronted pile of talus, as this is another rock glacier.

The trail soon curves west, enters sparse lodgepole forest, and, before long, trends south. You are now perched high above Charlotte Lake and have extensive views to the west: Charlotte Dome is the steep, polished dome downstream, and Mt. Bago is the large mountain at the southern end of Charlotte Lake. The summit of Mt. Bago provides the views to the Kings-Kern and Great Western divides that were lacking from Glen Pass. If you wish to summit Mt. Bago, take a detour at the Charlotte Lake junction a short ways downslope (see Appendix E). You continue your traverse and shortly reach a junction to Kearsarge Pass [10,760' – 2.0/2.0]. If you must exit to the Onion Valley Trailhead and the town of Independence to resupply, take this branch. Just a short distance downstream, you enter an enormous sandy flat, in the middle of which is the Charlotte Lake junction [10,740' – 0.3/2.3]. There is ample camping, a bear box, and a ranger station at the northeastern end of Charlotte Lake. Alternatively, heading east from this junction also takes you to Kearsarge Pass.

Leaving the sandy flat behind, you ascend briefly through white-bark and lodgepole pines, cross an exposed knob with foxtail pines, descend a short, steep slope with rocky footing, and reach yet another junction that leads to Kearsarge Pass—this one via Bullfrog Lake and

Location	Elevation	Distance from Previous Point	Cumulative Distance	UTM Coordinates
Glen Pass	11,960	—	0	11S 374134E 4072250N
Kearsarge Pass junction	10,760	2.0	2.0	11S 373529E 4070466N
Charlotte Lake junction	10,740	0.3	2.3	11S 373761E 4070152N
Bullfrog Lake junction	10,515	0.5	2.8	11S 374109E 4069881N
Bubbs Creek junction	9515	1.3	4.1	11S 374004E 4068999N
Upper Vidette Meadow bear box	9945	1.2	5.3	11S 375571E 4068228N
Center Basin Creek crossing	10,540	2.1	7.4	11S 377503E 4065728N
Lake at 12,250 feet	12,250	3.1	10.5	11S 377826E 4062513N
Forester Pass	13,100	1.3	11.8	11S 377385E 4061650N

SEE MAP 3

the Kearsarge Lakes Basin [10,515' – 0.5/2.8]. There is a small tent site near the junction, but camping is prohibited at Bullfrog Lake, and stock are prohibited on this trail. The JMT continues dropping south into the Bubbs Creek canyon. While the descent is mostly through steep, dry lodgepole forest, there are small, flat campsites near two creek crossings. At each of the stream crossings, you pass the expected collection of species: Coulter's daisy, great red paintbrush, Kelley's tiger lily, arrowleaf groundsel, corn lily, and swamp onion. Halfway down, where the trail briefly exits the forest, you are on a slope covered with bush chinquapin and are likely looking across the canyon to the steep face of East Vidette. There are large, shady campsites at the Bubbs Creek Trail junction [9515' – 1.3/4.1], where the Bubbs Creek Trail continues downstream to Roads End at Cedar Grove, while the JMT resumes its upward march.

The trail meanders along the flat, dry forest floor, crossing the outlet from Bullfrog Lake, a ford that can be a wade in early season. The forest is nearly barren—for long stretches, the upright pods of rock cress are all you see. You shortly pass Vidette Meadow, where there are large campsites and a bear box beneath lodgepole pines. There is also an excellent view of the east face of East Vidette. The trail briefly emerges onto a steeper, open slope, before leveling out near upper Vidette Meadow. Here, there are additional bear boxes and good campsites, both along the main creek and near the several tributaries you cross [9945' – 1.2/5.3]. Now the grade becomes gradual to moderate, and the forest cover thins as you ascend beside the wonderful cascades and pools of upper Bubbs Creek. For long stretches, the landscape is covered with downed tree limbs—evidence of past avalanches. Fireweed and low-growing willows are pioneer plants in this landscape. Due to this disturbance, your views are open; be sure to look up at the steep walls of East Vidette and southward to Center Peak. After this long stretch with limited camping options, you finally re-enter open lodgepole forest. Shortly thereafter, you pass a small cairn and note a conspicuous line of rocks indicating the start of the trail, the only remaining marker for the Center Basin Trail junction. Just beyond are large campsites and a bear box. A short distance later, you ford Center Basin Creek [10,540' – 2.1/7.4], which can be high in early season, and pass the last forested campsites for many miles.

You quickly leave the lodgepole forest behind. By now, you are familiar with the subalpine landscape: Scattered whitebark pines dot the landscape; where there are small streams, the ground is marshy and the vegetation includes mountaineer shooting stars, dwarf bilberry, little

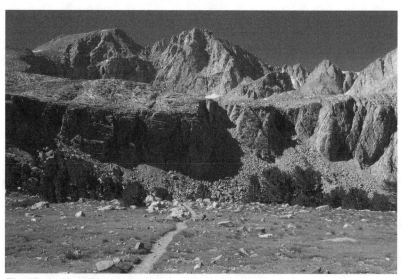

The Kings-Kern Divide viewed on the climb to Forester Pass

elephant's heads, Lemmon's paintbrush, and primrose monkeyflower; where you cross dry slabs or drier sedge meadows, Parish's yampah, pussytoes, and Sierra penstemon dominate. Above a series of small creeks, there are campsites on sandy, whitebark-pine-covered knobs, with spectacular views up and down Bubbs Creek: To the southwest is the vertical face of Mt. Stanford, and to the south is the steep Kings-Kern Divide. You pass more meadows, creeks, and, increasingly, piles of talus. This is the land of the alpine chipmunks and pikas. These small, round members of the rabbit family with adorable Mickey Mouse ears emit a two-noted *cheep-cheep* when disturbed. Most impressively, this species does not hibernate in winter, but lives beneath talus piles, eating piles of hay it has prepared in summer. At 11,230 feet, you pass the last clump of whitebark pines and another small campsite. There is another even more exposed campsite at the edge of the next meadow, with even more magnificent views, of course.

It is difficult to imagine that you have left the last tree behind, yet you still have nearly 2000 feet to climb to Forester Pass. As you continue your climb into the alpine zone, you will see occasional sandy tent spots among meadows and slabs. As always, please be sure to camp in previously used locations to limit your impact on resources in this fragile area. Moving rocks exposes the roots of the small alpine plants, causing them to desiccate and likely die. The JMT strikes east across an alpine meadow, near the shallow, gravelly Bubbs Creek. Then it climbs

SEE MAP 2

a short stretch of switchbacks and emerges on one last meadow and a slab-strewn bench. This landscape is the home of water pipets, spotted sandpipers, and gray-crowned rosy finches. Water pipets and spotted sandpipers are both especially common in Center Basin, to the east, with its expansive wet, hummocky, alpine meadows. If you are lucky, you may see a golden eagle soaring high above the mountains.

The remainder of the climb is now through talus, and here you will, for the first time on the JMT, see abundant specimens of the Sierra's two classic alpine species that are restricted to the highest elevation talus fields: sky pilot and alpine gold. Sky pilot has unmistakable 3-inch-diameter, deep purple heads of tubular flowers, and alpine gold is a yellow daisy with remarkably sticky stems and leaves. But probably most remarkable about these two is their size; in marked contrast to the fellfield species you have seen over the 12,000-foot passes, both of these plants are 4 to 8 inches tall. Shortly, you reach the outlet of Lake 12,250 (or 12,090 on older maps) [12,250' – 3.1/10.5]. Barren and stark, there are some small tent and bivy sites in the talus to the east of the outlet, with the potential for a beautiful sunset view of Junction Peak reflecting in the lake.

Just below the outlet, where the water mostly flows beneath the talus field, you cross the creek one last time, and climb to Forester Pass. You ascend a narrow ridge, enjoy your last views toward Mt. Stanford, and then commence the final southward traverse and ensuing switchbacks, where snow may linger very late. On the north side of this pass there are often no visible plants—most species cannot grow during the brief, snow-free weeks, and many others will emerge from rootstock only following the milder winters.

Forester Pass is atop the Kings-Kern Divide, the border between the Kings River drainage that you have been traversing since Muir Pass, and the Kern River drainage to the south. While the Kings River has many east-west trending forks, resulting in one high pass after another, the Kern River runs north-south and therefore the next stretch of the JMT has fewer long descents and ascents. Instead, you find yourself climbing in and out of many small canyons and then, of course, up the slopes of Mt. Whitney. This high pass is also the border between Kings Canyon and Sequoia national parks. And a word of warning: Enjoy the views from the north side of the pass, as the south side is quite a wind funnel [13,100' – 1.3/11.8]!

SEE MAP 2

SECTION 12.

Forester Pass to
Trail Crest—Kern River

The view from the top of Forester Pass is breathtaking and vast: To the southwest are the dark, jagged summits of the Kaweahs; to their east, the long, straight fault scarp through which flows the Kern River; and straight ahead, the magnificent rolling tundra landscape through which you will shortly walk. As you next stare down the steep southern side of Forester Pass, you will not be surprised that trail engineers had initially planned to route the JMT elsewhere. A circuitous route was first constructed through Center Basin, then across Junction Pass, taking hikers east of the crest, and finally back across Shepherd Pass, to merge again with the current JMT route near the Tyndall Creek crossing. However, by 1931, the route over Forester Pass was discovered, scouted, and built, streamlining the route south to Whitney. In winter, however, skiers still use creative route-finding to successfully cross this divide. Now

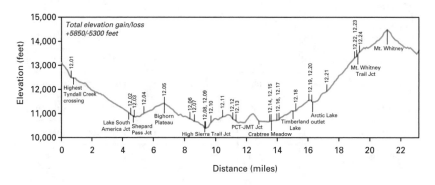

SEE MAP 2

you descend numerous exposed switchbacks, some of which are cut into the rock, and others of which are built atop stone walls. Growing on this near-vertical cliff face are club-moss ivesia, as always, sticking out from cracks. A bit lower is abundant magenta-colored, four-petal rockfringe, growing from the base of boulders and outcrops. Where the grade eases are small, very exposed, and austere sandy patches that fit a small tent. Just thereafter, you cross the nascent Tyndall Creek for the first time [12,480' – 0.8/0.8].

You now begin a delightful walk down the broad, gentle valley. To the east, the steep faces of Junction Peak and Diamond Mesa are incongruous. The summits of these peaks were never glaciated, and the steep, smooth chutes on their western faces are all the result of ava-

Location	Elevation	Distance from Previous Point	Cumulative Distance	UTM Coordinates
Forester Pass	13,100	—	0	11S 377385E 4061650N
Highest Tyndall Creek crossing	12,480	0.8	0.8	11S 377187E 4061065N
Lake South America junction	11,050	3.6	4.4	11S 375989E 4056214N
Shepherd Pass junction	10,890	0.3	4.7	11S 376038E 4055756N
Bighorn Plateau	11,415	2.0	6.7	11S 376718E 4053197N
Wright Creek crossing	10,700	1.9	8.6	11S 377120E 4051003N
High Sierra Trail junction	10,405	0.7	9.3	11S 377431E 4050545N
Ridge west of Mt. Young	10,963	1.5	10.8	11S 377128E 4048924N
PCT junction west of Crabtree Meadows	10,700	2.0	12.8	11S 378224E 4046604N
Crabtree Meadow and ranger station	10,700	0.8	13.6	11S 379242E 4047254N
Timberline Lake outlet	11,090	1.4	15.0	11S 380984E 4047519N
Arctic Lake outlet creek	11,480	1.3	16.3	11S 382571E 4048021N
Mt. Whitney Trail junction	13,450	2.9	19.2	11S 384365E 4046710N
Mt. Whitney	14,505	1.9	21.1	11S 384474E 4048692N
Trail Crest	13,650	2.1	23.2	11S 384501E 4046570N

SEE MAP 2

lanche activity; only the lower reaches of the peaks bear signs of past glaciation. For many miles, you wander through this sandy landscape, dotted by boulders and alpine tarns of all sizes, and with abundant fellfield species covering the ground. Three different species of buckwheat share this area: the yellow-flowered frosted buckwheat that has been common on all dry substrates from the montane to the alpine; the white- to pink-flowered, oval-leaved buckwheat, which bears such dense hairs that they appear nearly white; and foxtail buckwheat, a yellow-flowered species with spade-shaped leaves and long flower stalks lying horizontally on the ground. Growing so close to the ground allows these plants to avoid the persistent wind chill and to maintain leaf temperatures warmer than the surrounding air. Where the trail becomes just a bit steeper is the departure point for a side trip up Caltech Peak. From that summit, you will be able to look straight into the Lake South America Basin and at the Kings-Kern Divide (see Appendix E). Lower down, you skirt the creeks and meadows, as the trail has been rerouted in places to avoid damage to the streamside vegetation. In the distance, you get your first view of Mt. Whitney, the tall, flat-topped peak with large avalanche chutes on its northern face.

The trail passes through one small stand of mixed lodgepole and foxtail pines and shortly reaches a signed junction for the now unmaintained Lake South America Trail, taking you to the true headwaters of the Kern River, and a beautiful basin to explore if time permits [11,050′ – 3.6/4.4]. A short distance later, you reach the Tyndall Creek crossing and camping area (with bear box); please camp in the locations specified by the ranger and note that campfires are prohibited within 1200 feet of the crossing. This creek crossing may be short, but the fast-flowing, freezing-cold water and rocky bottom makes it formidable in early season. In a few more steps, you pass the Shepherd Pass Trail, the Sequoia National Park side of which has been newly rebuilt to skirt the marshy areas in the valley [10,890′ – 0.3/4.7]. Next, you pass a junction for the trail that heads down Tyndall Creek. The Tyndall Creek ranger station is a good distance down this trail (about 0.7 mile)—much farther than is shown on many maps. There are campsites at the junction. Now you can avoid navigating for a number of miles: Head south (left) and uphill, following zigzags toward the Tyndall Frog Ponds where there are large campsites, a bear box, and warmish swimming. Again, campfires are prohibited within 1200 feet of the camping area. There are beautiful views of Diamond Mesa from the ponds.

You continue climbing, skirting around the western side of Tawny Point, first through dry lodgepole forest, then onto drier, more exposed

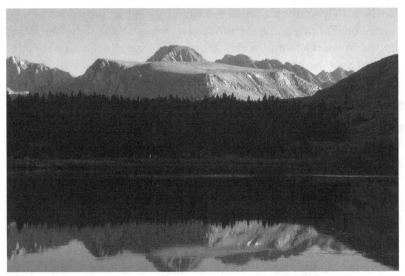

Diamond Mesa and Junction Peak viewed from the Tyndall Frog Ponds

slopes that are dominated by foxtail pines, and eventually onto a barren landscape of sandy ground broken only by tufts of sedges. The views keep opening up; not only can you see the country you have just traversed to the north, but also ever more of the Great Western Divide. From south to north are Milestone Mountain, a narrow pinnacle; Midway Mountain, a not-too-inspiring peak; Table Mountain, with vertical sides and a flat top; and Thunder Mountain, a steep and imposing pyramid. Where the trail crests is a nearly round tarn [11,415' – 2.0/6.7]. This is Bighorn Plateau, named for sheep once seen in the area. Ironically, the plateau itself is lousy sheep habitat, as the sheep stick to cliffy areas where they can outmaneuver predators. Sandy, flat, unvegetated patches make for possible campsites, and their views speak for themselves. But even if you don't spend a night here, plan ahead to spend some time, as the location is magical: Early in the morning, you'll likely hear packs of coyotes; a few hours later, you can watch the ravens sitting in the foxtail pine snags; American kestrels and other birds of prey will soar above you; and marmots will sun themselves on nearby boulders. In case the view isn't quite good enough, climb up Tawny Point for the full panorama (see Appendix E), or wander westward to one of the shorter knobs overlooking the Kern drainage.

After Bighorn Plateau, the JMT descends into the Wright Creek drainage. A hardscrabble sandy slope marks the remnants of an old moraine. Elsewhere, the trail skirts the top of long meadows with small

SEE MAP 1

streams, tributaries of Wright Creek, filled with Bigelow's sneezeweed, a wild sunflower with big, bright, yellow flowers and dark "noses." A few campsites present themselves as you drop into lodgepole forest, and you'll encounter a much better one just after you ford the main Wright Creek. This crossing may be difficult in early season, as the water can be deep [10,700' – 1.9/8.6]. Another short climb follows, and you cross a forested flat, reach the lip of the Wallace Creek drainage, enjoy yet another vista to the Kaweahs, and descend on a dry, sandy slope to the High Sierra Trail junction [10,405' – 0.7/9.3], which goes west to the Giant Forest. Just beyond the junction is the Wallace Creek crossing, which can also be difficult in early season, for although the rocks underfoot are small, it is a long crossing. On the south bank are popular campsites and a bear box. Note that, once again, campfires are not permitted within 1200 feet of the bear box.

Yet again, the JMT heads uphill, this time skirting around the giant west shoulder of Mt. Young, en route to Crabtree Meadow. The climb begins in lodgepole forest, but as soon as the slope gets steeper, foxtail pines become dominant. As you ascend, note that the granite you pass is pinkish, due to potassium feldspar, one of the minerals in granite. Here it is easily visible, as the granite has a greater percent of potassium feldspar, and the individual rectangular crystals are large. Elsewhere, note greenish surfaces on fractured boulders; this is the mineral epidote, which commonly fills small cracks in granite. Where the slope eases, the foxtail pines again give way to lodgepoles, as the two species thrive in slightly different environments. Shortly, you cross a creek, beside which is one small tent site, and you continue upward through moister terrain. The JMT crosses several other small trickles and climbs up through an open forest of foxtail pines and huge boulders to the apex of the shoulder [10,963' – 1.5/10.8]. When water is available, sandy patches would make elegant campsites offering artistic pine trees and a filtered view across to the Kaweah Peaks. The ensuing traverse and slight descent leads to the edge of Sandy Meadow, which the JMT skirts along its upper edge. Where you first reach the meadow, there are large campsites a bit to the west, the direction of the old trail. The forest floor is bare, save scattered individuals of a few species, including foxtail buckwheat, Sierra penstemon, and Nuttall's sandwort. But the banks of each little trickle you cross are densely covered, and here you find primrose monkeyflower, carpet clover, Parish's yampah, ranger's buttons, and much more. Hopefully you are not yet too tired of this lumpy topography, as there is one more ascent ahead, up to a ridge radiating southwest from Mt. Young, followed by a descent to a trail

SEE MAP 1

junction, where the PCT and JMT part company for good. The PCT continues south from here to the Mexican border, but you turn eastward for your last ascent of the trip: up nearly 4000 feet to the summit of Mt. Whitney [10,700' – 2.0/12.8].

The JMT heads east, along a dry bench with scattered foxtail pines, staying above Whitney Creek's north bank. At times, the summit of Mt. Whitney is visible through the trees. Shortly after you enter denser forest cover, pass one campsite, and ascend a zigzag, you reach the Crabtree junction [10,700' – 0.8/13.6]. Turning right takes you to the Crabtree ranger station, a bear box, and a selection of campsites. Mt. Whitney is straight ahead. Also at this junction is a large box containing human waste bags that all hikers bound for Whitney Portal are required to use east of Crabtree Meadows. Please take one and preserve the water quality for all future hikers (see the introductory section on water purification and camp hygiene on page 20 for additional information).

You continue upward along the north shore of Whitney Creek, on a river terrace, first through open lodgepole forest, passing several campsites, and then increasingly across dry, open slopes. The latter are covered with shaggy hawkweed, small-leaved cream bush, wavy-leaved paintbrush, pennyroyal, granite gilia, and, for the first time since Thousand Island Lake, the periwinkle-colored western blue flax. A stemless white thistle is elk thistle, and the yellow-rayed daisy with non-hairy serrate leaves is Fremont's groundsel. A set of switchbacks up slabs take you to Timberline Lake [11,090' – 1.4/15.0], where camping is prohibited, but photographing Mt. Whitney mirrored in its still waters is encouraged. Shortly, you'll pass one small campsite, nestled among willows above Timberline Lake. As your climb continues, to your left is a dry, sandy slope, and to your right is various meadow and creekside vegetation. Beneath rocks is pink heuchera and occasionally Sierra primrose and rockfringe, while red mountain heather covers large expanses of sandy substrate, doing a remarkable job of holding the loose material in place. When the trail levels out into a wet-sandy flat, you are nearly at Guitar Lake. Here, you can leave the trail to find campsites above the "guitar's neck," or you can continue up the trail and across Arctic Lake's outlet [11,480' – 1.3/16.3] to additional camping. All sites have beautiful views of the evening alpenglow on the west, now hulking, face of Mt. Whitney and good morning light in the direction of the Kaweahs. Be sure to fill your water bottles here, as in some years, it is the last water until Trail Camp, nearly 10 miles away on the other side of Mt. Whitney.

SEE MAP 1

After skirting the meadow at the inlet of Guitar Lake and passing two small tarns, your final 3000-foot (!) climb begins. You first climb up sandy, bouldery slopes, crisscrossed by seeps, many of which are filled with Bigelow's sneezeweed. Just below 12,000 feet, you reach a bench, dotted with small seasonal ponds and edged with slabs. There are fantastic views from this bench down to the Hitchcock Lakes, across to Mt. Hitchcock, and, of course, expansive views westward. And on the slabs, a short distance west of the trail, are your last large campsites before Mt. Whitney. Now you find yourself on endless switchbacks in increasingly barren talus. You'll notice that the granite here is very light colored—there are few dark crystals—and that the rock contains large, rectangular feldspar crystals. If you're lucky, you'll see ones embedded with dark, rectangular outlines of minuscule dark minerals, showing where other minerals began to grow but were engulfed by a single, ever-expanding feldspar crystal. Upward you climb, now in the realm of the rosy finches and ravens. Sky pilot and alpine gold are abundant here, joined by a few other hardy species such as Sierra primrose, rock-fringe, Fremont's groundsel, granite draba, mountain sorrel, club-moss ivesia, Sierra fleabane daisy, and another daisy with three-lobed leaves, Sierra cutleaf daisy. Sometimes its central yellow disc is rimmed by purple ray petals, and other times these are absent. The higher you go, the fewer species you find growing, until only sky pilot and alpine gold are common. As you finally approach the Mt. Whitney Trail junction, you note a few austere bivy and small tent sites, where boulders have been used to build small walls and the sandy area in between can hold a small tent. Suddenly, you reach the trail junction [13,450′ – 2.9/19.2] and intersect the vast quantities of human traffic headed for Mt. Whitney's summit: On most summer days, 150 people have received either a day-use or overnight permit to ascend the peak from Whitney Portal.

Most JMT hikers leave their overnight packs (or at least most of its contents) at this location, carrying only water, food, a jacket, and, of course, a camera, to the summit. Although you are well-acclimated, take these last miles slowly. Don't push yourself so hard that you need constant breaks, but instead find a pace that allows you to keep oxygen intake in balance with exertion. You climb first up a talus slope, passing additional campsites right on the Sierra Crest. For a long stretch, the trail then winds past notch-like windows and among pinnacles, the tallest of which is Class 3-4 Mt. Muir, another 14,000-foot peak. It is a beautiful peak and an exhilarating climb, but didn't John Muir deserve more than a subsidiary peak of that named for his nemesis, Josiah Whitney? The trail then emerges on one final giant, barren, talus slope, and

SEE MAP 1

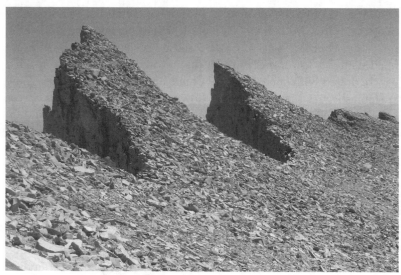

Pinnacles south of Mt. Whitney

passes two even taller, but much less steep pinnacles, Day Needle and Keeler Needle, which are considered insufficiently distinct from Mt. Whitney to be called "peaks." Now you complete the final switchbacks to the summit, arriving at the metal-roofed summit building and the enormous summit register [14,505' – 1.9/21.1]. From there, you will undoubtedly head east to the true summit, marked by a metal plaque. Unless a storm threatens, give yourself a good long break on top—you have just completed the JMT! Walk around the entire summit plateau, as there is a unique view in each direction. Especially stunning is to look down the east face of the mountain, to Trail Camp and Consultation Lake, and beyond to the town of Lone Pine, 10,000 feet below. The end of your trip lies some 5000 feet below, so retrace your steps to the junction and turn east, leaving the official JMT, for 0.1 more mile to the highest pass on this journey, Trail Crest [13,650' – 2.1/23.2].

SEE MAP 1

SECTION 13.

Trail Crest to Whitney Portal—Owens River

At Trail Crest, you leave Sequoia National Park and enter John Muir Wilderness. You are now in the Lone Pine Creek drainage, which flows into the Owens River, dead-ending in Owens Lake. You are once again on a steep, talus slope, this one laced with just under 100 tight switchbacks; back and forth you go down the northeast-facing slope. About two-thirds of the way down is a section where the trail has been blasted into a cliff. Here, water seeps through cracks, and this section is notorious for being ice-covered most of the time. Fortunately, there is a cable you can cling to if necessary. The grueling descent ends at Trail Camp [12,040' – 2.3/2.3]. Tent sites have been created in every flat spot available among the pervasive slabs and boulders, and there are many places to camp on both sides of the trail. The solar toilet that was once

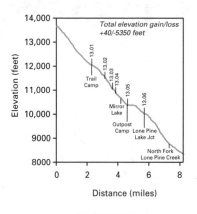

here was closed in 2006, so be sure to use the waste bag you picked up at the Crabtree junction. Unfortunately, the only thing missing from your alpine perch is a good view of the east face of Mt. Whitney; the rock glacier rising straight above camp blocks the view of Mt. Whitney, which is a good deal north of you. This can be remedied by an early-morning ascent of Wotans Throne, the peak immediately south of Trail Camp that is best climbed from its northern or northwestern side (see Appendix E). I advocate a predawn start, so that you can watch the sunrise on Mt. Whitney's east face. After nearly completing your journey, this may not sound appealing, but after 40 other campers and many dayhikers start tromping around and through camp in the wee hours, why not get up and enjoy the morning light?

You now have just 6 miles to go! You descend a granite trail, crossing Lone Pine Creek, and passing now familiar flowers such as rockfringe, alpine prickly currant, small-leaved cream bush, granite gilia, and clubmoss ivesia. The thornless currant is the wax (or squaw) currant, and is likewise abundant. Along rock faces is cliff bush, under rocks is Sierra primrose, and where it's wetter are the mountain and primrose monkeyflowers. You pass one small campsite just before you reach a small, wet meadow (camping prohibited), through which Lone Pine Creek flows. This area is filled with brightly colored mountaineer shooting stars. The first trees appear around 11,000 feet, at which point there are simultaneously stunted foxtail pine and lodgepole pine. Some switchbacks later, and past a few small and potentially dry campsites, the trail finally flattens out at Mirror Lake, where camping is prohibited [10,630' – 1.9/4.2]. You cross its outlet and proceed downward, across a dry, south-facing

Location	Elevation	Distance from Previous Point	Cumulative Distance	UTM Coordinates
Trail Crest	13,650	—	0	11S 384501E 4046570N
Trail Camp	12,040	2.3	2.3	11S 385618E 4046947N
Mirror Lake	10,630	1.9	4.2	11S 387198E 4047790N
Outpost Camp	10,370	0.4	4.6	11S 387479E 4047910N
Lone Pine Lake junction	9990	1.1	5.7	11S 388234E 4048294N
North Fork Lone Pine Creek crossing	8730	1.6	7.3	11S 388673E 4049564N
Whitney Portal	8330	0.9	8.2	11S 389173E 4049571N

SEE MAP 1

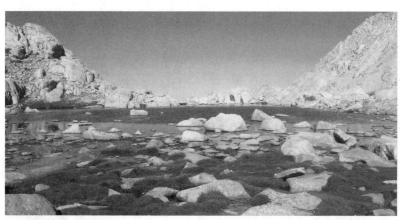

Lake at Trail Camp

slope covered with bush chinquapin, wavy-leaved paintbrush, penny-royal, shaggy hawkweed, mountain pride penstemon, and scarlet penstemon. At the bottom of the slope lies Outpost Camp [10,370' – 0.4/4.6], a second large camping area beneath tall foxtail pines. The toilet once here also has been closed. The trail curves southeast along the upper edge of the adjacent marshy area, Bighorn Park. Leaving this area, you climb slightly before descending switchbacks to a large, sandy flat covered with mousetail ivesia. Here you'll spot the sign marking the end of the Mt. Whitney Zone. Around the corner is the lateral to Lone Pine Lake, at which there are campsites [9990' – 1.1/5.7].

From here, you have only 2.5 miles to go. But as you race downward, take time to look at the steep, white granite walls on either side of the canyon and the view down Lone Pine Creek. You descend through open lodgepole forest to a log crossing over Lone Pine Creek. Shortly, your exposed descent continues down yet another set of seemingly endless switchbacks. The lower you get, the less familiar the vegetation is; for the first time on your journey, you encounter the mid-elevation, dry, eastside chaparral community: mountain mahogany, with its white, twisted "seed-tails" and inrolled leaves; single-leaf pinyon pine; fernbush, a tall shrub with fern-like leaves and white flowers; and Rothrock's beardtongue, a light pink relative of the penstemons. You shortly cross the main branch of the North Fork of Lone Pine Creek [8730' – 1.6/7.3], which can be difficult early season, as well as a small tributary, and then walk your final mile to Whitney Portal, where you can weigh your now nearly empty backpack [8330' – 0.9/8.2]. Congratulations, you've made it!

SEE MAP 1

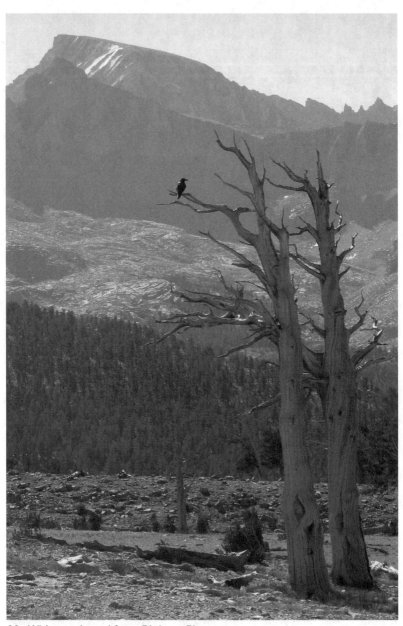

Mt. Whitney viewed from Bighorn Plateau

SOUTH TO NORTH:
WHITNEY PORTAL TO YOSEMITE VALLEY

SECTION 13.

Whitney Portal to
Trail Crest—Owens River

You will probably begin your trip by reading the panels at the trail-head and weighing your pack on the handy scale—undoubtedly deciding that your hiking companions should be taking some of your weight! You begin by switchbacking up a sandy, south-facing slope, covered with drought-tolerant shrubs and herbs that are members of the eastside chaparral community. Among others are mountain mahogany, with its white, twisted "seed-tails" and in-rolled leaves; single-leaf pinyon pine; fernbush, a tall shrub with fern-like leaves and white flowers; and Rothrock's beardtongue, with light pink, tubular flowers. The next miles are the only section of the JMT where you will see these species. Shortly, you reach a small tributary and just thereafter the main branch of the North Fork of Lone Pine Creek [8730' – 0.9/0.9].

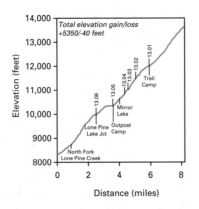

SEE MAP 1

The trail now changes to an east aspect and climbs up many sandy switchbacks. Be sure to stop, turn around, and look at the steep, white granite walls on either side of the canyon, as well as the view down Lone Pine Creek. This is the only view you'll have of the expansive and barren eastern Sierra. One bird you might see hopping in and out of the scrubby vegetation is the fox sparrow. These brown, slightly streaked sparrows are a bit larger than other sparrows with which you may be familiar. As you climb, a few taller trees begin to mingle with the dry scrub. The first is white fir, with longish needles attached individually to branches; this is a species you will see only where the JMT drops below 9000 feet. Higher still, you find yourself beneath the first towering Jeffrey pines, with long needles in clusters of three, and large cones. These trees usually stand on their own in drier and rockier areas, rather than forming continuous forest cover. Among the overwhelming diversity of small plants is one with tall stems bearing red, tubular flowers; this is scarlet penstemon, which will greet you on dry slopes throughout your walk. Where the grade eases, you hike through some wetter vegetation and then on logs across Lone Pine Creek, although getting to the logs can be wet when the water is high.

Across the stream, you enter an open forest, a near monostand of lodgepole pine, the species that will dominate along much of the trail. Lodgepole pines are characterized by small, round cones that are always abundant around tree trunks, needles in clusters of two, and fine-scaly bark. Around the corner is the lateral to Lone Pine Lake, at which there are campsites [9990' – 1.6/2.5]. You next cross a sandy flat, with a sign that you are entering the Mt. Whitney Zone, and proceed

Location	Elevation	Distance from Previous Point	Cumulative Distance	UTM Coordinates
Whitney Portal	8330	—	0	11S 389173E 4049571N
North Fork Lone Pine Creek crossing	8730	0.9	0.9	11S 388673E 4049564N
Lone Pine Lake junction	9990	1.6	2.5	11S 388234E 4048294N
Outpost Camp	10,370	1.1	3.6	11S 387479E 4047910N
Mirror Lake	10,630	0.4	4.0	11S 387198E 4047790N
Trail Camp	12,040	1.9	5.9	11S 385618E 4046947N
Trail Crest	13,650	2.3	8.2	11S 384501E 4046570N

SEE MAP 1

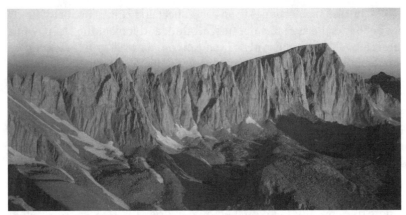

Sunrise over Mt. Whitney (the peak on the far right)

up yet more switchbacks. You have now left the chaparral community, and the plants present on this slope are also present west of the crest. One you will see again and again is small-leaved cream bush, a shrub that boasts white, five-petal flowers on pinkish stems and small serrate leaves. At the top of the slope, the trail drops slightly and skirts around the southern edge of a marshy area, Bighorn Park. At the far western edge of this flat is Outpost Camp [10,370' – 1.1/3.6], a large camping area beneath tall foxtail pines. This is a southern Sierra species that will disappear as you head north. Their long, dangling branches often have needles only near the tip, where they encircle the stem like a bottle-brush. The solar toilet that used to be here was closed in 2006 because its composting mechanism cannot keep up with the heavy use. As a JMT hiker starting at Whitney Portal, you are one of the few people on the trail not required to pack out your human waste (though this may change in the future). Nonetheless, please be cognizant that the incredibly heavy human impacts in this area necessitate that you be especially careful to bury your waste far from campsites and water sources. (See the introductory section on water quality and camp hygiene on page 20 for additional information.)

You have now climbed 2000 feet, but still have a long way to go. The next set of switchbacks are again on a dry, south-facing slope. Bush chinquapin, a relative of oaks, is the dominant shrub here. It is easily identified by its spiny fruit and leathery leaves, whose undersides are gold-colored. Two common herbs are pennyroyal, an aromatic mint with a head of small, purple flowers, and wavy-leaved paintbrush. The paintbrush sports a dense head of red-orange tubular flowers whose ends are pointed or beaked. You will encounter many paintbrushes

SEE MAP 1

along the JMT, and this one is distinguished by its wavy-margined leaves. At the top of this slope, you reach Mirror Lake, where camping is prohibited, and cross its outlet [10,630′ – 0.4/4.0].

The trail now ascends a north-facing slope beneath big foxtail pines. On a few small benches are established campsites, but they are far from water. Another timberline tree species occurs sporadically here, the whitebark pine. This tree, with needles in clusters of five, can occur up to 12,000 feet in places, forming krumholz, the German name referring to the stunted and twisted trees at the highest elevations. And just a bit higher, you leave the last tree behind: Until you are west of Mt. Whitney, you are in the alpine zone. The sandy trail continues up amongst slabs and the views keep opening up. Alongside slabs grow two species of currants: The thornless currant is the wax (or squaw) currant, and the thornier, and concurrently tastier, species is the alpine prickly currant. The latter is common not only in the alpine zone, but also as a sprawling ground cover in many lodgepole forests.

Shortly, you reach a small, wet meadow (camping prohibited), through which Lone Pine Creek flows. The meadow is filled with brightly colored mountaineer shooting stars. A short distance up is one small campsite, nestled on a sandy platform among slabs. The colorful flowers keep dazzling your eyes. Beneath rocks is the bright pink Sierra primrose, a high-elevation southern Sierra species that will follow you only half way to Yosemite. Along rock faces is cliff bush, a pink-flowered shrub whose stems emerge from cracks and whose branches literally hug the rock. In seeps are the large, yellow, tubular flowers belonging to the mountain monkeyflower. Distracted by the plants, the interminable switchbacks go just a bit faster en route to Trail Camp [12,040′ – 1.9/5.9]. Tent sites have been created in every flat spot available among the pervasive slabs and boulders, and there are many places to camp on both sides of the trail. The toilet here has also been closed, so be sure to find a "toilet" well away from the crowded camping area. (Note that the toilet has also been removed from the summit of Mt. Whitney.)

Most hikers who camp here are anxious to get an early start up to the summit of Mt. Whitney, an especially good idea if you are even slightly uncertain about the afternoon weather. But should you be especially masochistic, you may choose to take an early-morning detour up Wotans Throne, the peak immediately south of Trail Camp that is best climbed from its northern or northwestern side (see Appendix E). Watching the sunrise on Mt. Whitney's east face from this vantage point is outstanding.

SEE MAP 1

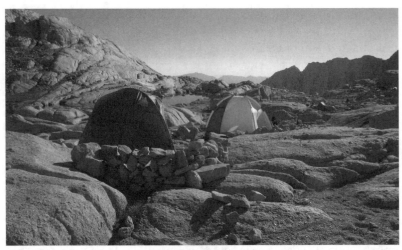

Trail Camp

Detour or not, you will shortly be joining the crowd of people ascending the switchbacks up to Trail Crest, the pass leading to the west side of the crest. The talus slope in front of you is laced with just under 100 tight switchbacks; back and forth you go, ascending the northeast-facing slope. About one third of the way up is a section notorious for being ice-covered most of the time. Fortunately, there is a cable you can cling too if necessary. This talus slope looks unbelievably barren from a distance, but if you stare at your feet (as happens all too easily while walking uphill) you will see a continuous flow of plants passing by. Two of the most common ones, sky pilot and alpine gold, which will follow you nearly to the summit of Whitney, are abundant only here and while crossing Forester Pass, for farther north the passes are too low. Sky pilot has unmistakable 3-inch-diameter, deep purple heads of tubular flowers, and alpine gold is a yellow daisy with remarkably sticky stems and leaves. But probably most remarkable about these two is their size: Both of these plants are 4 to 8 inches tall, much higher than most fellfield species you will encounter. Two other species might also engage your eye as your puff upwards: Mountain sorrel grows beneath shaded boulders and is identified by its rounded leaves and elongate stalks of either white flowers or red seeds. Granite (or Lemmon's) draba is a cushion plant that is ubiquitous under moist boulders. It is a type of mustard with small, four-petal, yellow flowers that cover the top of the cushion when in bloom. Finally, you reach the top of Trail Crest, more than 5000 feet above your starting point, and look down to the western slope of the Sierra [13,650' – 2.3/8.2].

SEE MAP 1

SECTION 12.

Trail Crest to
Forester Pass—Kern River

You continue along the Mt. Whitney Trail for 0.2 mile to intersect the JMT itself, 1.9 miles below the summit of Mt. Whitney. Most JMT hikers leave their overnight packs (or at least most of its contents) at this location, carrying only water, food, a jacket, and, of course, a camera, to the summit. Since you have not been at high elevation for long, take these last miles very slowly. Don't push yourself so hard that you need constant breaks. Instead, find a pace that allows you to keep oxygen intake in balance with exertion—slow and steady really does win the race!

You climb first up a talus slope, passing small campsites right on the Sierra Crest. Boulders have been used to build small walls around sandy patches large enough to hold a small tent. For a long stretch, the trail winds past notch-like windows and among pinnacles, the tallest of

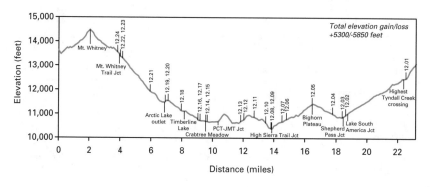

SEE MAP 1

which is Class 3-4 Mt. Muir, another 14,000-foot peak. This is a beautiful peak and an exhilarating climb, but didn't John Muir deserve more than a subsidiary peak of that named for his nemesis, Josiah Whitney? (Whitney was the state geologist who contested Muir's analysis that there was widespread evidence of past glaciation in the Sierra Nevada.) The trail then emerges on one final, giant, barren, talus slope, and passes two even taller (but much less steep) pinnacles, Day Needle and Keeler Needle, which are considered insufficiently distinct from Mt. Whitney to be called "peaks." Now you complete the final switchbacks to the top, arriving at the metal-roofed summit building and the enormous summit register [14,505' − 2.1/2.1]. From there, you will undoubtedly head east to the true summit, marked by a metal plaque. Unless a storm

Location	Elevation	Distance from Previous Point	Cumulative Distance	UTM Coordinates
Trail Crest	13,650	—	0	11S 384501E 4046570N
Mt. Whitney	14,505	2.1	2.1	11S 384474E 4048692N
Mt. Whitney Trail junction	13,450	1.9	4.0	11S 384365E 4046710N
Arctic Lake outlet creek	11,480	2.9	6.9	11S 382571E 4048021N
Timberline Lake outlet	11,090	1.3	8.2	11S 380984E 4047519N
Crabtree Meadow and ranger station	10,700	1.4	9.6	11S 379242E 4047254N
PCT junction west of Crabtree Meadows	10,760	0.8	10.4	11S 378224E 4046604N
Ridge west of Mt. Young	10,963	2.0	12.4	11S 377128E 4048924N
High Sierra Trail junction	10,405	1.5	13.9	11S 377431E 4050545N
Wright Creek crossing	10,700	0.7	14.6	11S 377120E 4051003N
Bighorn Plateau	11,415	1.9	16.5	11S 376718E 4053197N
Shepherd Pass junction	10,890	2.0	18.5	11S 376038E 4055756N
Lake South America junction	11,050	0.3	18.8	11S 375989E 4056214N
Highest Tyndall Creek crossing	12,480	3.6	22.4	11S 377187E 4061065N
Forester Pass	13,100	0.8	23.2	11S 377385E 4061650N

SEE MAP 1

threatens, give yourself a good, long break on top. Walk around the entire summit plateau, as there is a unique and magnificent view in each direction. Especially stunning is the view down the east face of the mountain to Trail Camp and Consultation Lake, and beyond to the town of Lone Pine, 10,000 feet below. Looking northwest, you can see the next stretch of the JMT, up over Bighorn Plateau, marked by a perfectly round tarn, and toward Forester Pass. Finally, pull yourself away from the views and retrace your steps to your pack [13,450' – 1.9/4.0].

Now leaving behind the crowds of people, you part ways with the Mt. Whitney Trail and begin the route north along the JMT, beginning with a 2000-foot descent to Guitar Lake. Above the first switchback, there are a few more austere bivy and small tent sites. At this elevation, only sky pilot and alpine gold are common. Ravens may fly overhead, and small flocks of gray-crowned rosy finches may pass by in search of insects, but mostly you are alone with the talus. If you look closely at the rocks, you'll notice that the granite here is very light—there are few dark crystals—and the rock contains large, rectangular feldspar crystals. If you're lucky, you'll see ones embedded with dark, rectangular outlines of minuscule dark minerals, showing where other minerals began to grow, but were engulfed by a single, ever-expanding feldspar crystal, a phenomena creating a "zoned" crystal. The view is spectacular: To the west are the dark, jagged Kaweah Peaks, and directly to the southwest is the steep face of Mt. Hitchcock. The gullies on the face are avalanche chutes, whose exact locations are determined by the location of joints within the granite. The rock in the joints is more easily fractured and displaced by freeze-thaw activity, and the loose rock is then carried downslope by the snow. In many places in the Sierra, these avalanches not only remove rock, but also polish the chutes.

As you slowly drop lower, additional plants appear. You'll again see the granite draba, mountain sorrel, and Sierra primrose present on the eastern escarpment. Two daisies may also catch your attention: Sierra fleabane daisy has long, fairly skinny leaves and a dense head of up to 120 purple ray petals that attach to a central yellow disc. In comparison, Sierra cutleaf daisy has three-lobed leaves, while its central yellow disc is rimmed by fewer white to purple ray petals that are sometimes altogether absent. In cracks in slabs emerge clumps of stalks topped by tufts of yellow flowers. These are club-moss ivesia, which are one of the dominant species at the highest elevations, always emerging from such cracks.

Just below 12,000 feet, you reach a bench dotted with small, seasonal ponds and edged with slabs. There are fantastic views from this bench down to the Hitchcock Lakes and across to Mt. Hitchcock, and, of course, expansive views westward. On the slabs a short distance west of the trail are beautiful campsites. You continue descending sandy, bouldery slopes, crisscrossed by seeps, pass two small tarns, and skirt around the meadow extending west from Guitar Lake's inlet. Shortly, you begin passing many small campsites. All have beautiful views of the evening alpenglow on the west, hulking, face of Mt. Whitney, and good morning light in the direction of the Kaweahs. If you leave the trail and head west along Guitar Lake's outlet, you will find additional campsites on the bluffs above the "guitar's neck." The trail crosses Arctic Lake's outlet stream [11,480' – 2.9/6.9], ascends slightly, and continues its downward trajectory. On your right is a dry, sandy slope, often covered in a sprawling plant with pink flowers and needle-like leaves. This is red mountain heather, a common species throughout the Sierra from the montane to the alpine zones, and one that does a remarkable job of holding loose material in place. Beneath rocks you may find Sierra primrose, but also rockfringe, a species with even bigger, four-petal magenta flowers, or pink huechera, a species with small, light pink, bell-shaped flowers, and round, lobed leaves. In the wet meadows alongside small creeks grow mountaineer shooting star and Bigelow's sneezeweed, a wild sunflower with big, bright, yellow ray petals and dark "noses." As you approach Timberline Lake, you pass one small campsite nestled among willows. Camping is prohibited at Timberline Lake [11,090' – 1.3/8.2], but photographing Mt. Whitney mirrored in its still waters is encouraged.

You descend a few switchbacks, skirt a small meadow, and once again continue across dry, open slopes covered with small-leaved cream bush, wavy-leaved paintbrush, pennyroyal, and much more. You may also see the stemless white elk thistle; Anderson's thistle, with bright red or magenta flowers on tall stalks; and Fremont's groundsel, a yellow-rayed daisy with non-hairy serrate leaves. My favorite is the periwinkle-colored western blue flax, which you will not see again until you are north of Devils Postpile. Shortly, you drop into open lodgepole forest, passing several campsites along the north shore of Whitney Creek, and then reach the Crabtree junction [10,700' – 1.4/9.6]. Turn right to reach the Crabtree ranger station, a bear box, and a selection of campsites. You descend a zigzag, pass one more campsite, for a short distance continue through lodgepole forest, and then emerge on a dry bench with scattered foxtail pines, staying above Whitney Creek's north bank. A slight ascent takes you to another junction, this one where the Pacific Crest Trail and the JMT merge [10,700' – 0.8/10.4]. The two

SEE MAP 1

trails will now follow the same path for most of the route north to Tuolumne Meadows.

Now begins a long section of "lumpy" topography: There are no particularly long ascents or descents, yet you are constantly traversing shoulders that radiate west from some peak, and then dropping into another small drainage. Your first climb is up a ridge extending southwest of Mt. Young. Down the backside, you begin a long traverse above and around Sandy Meadow. Much of your walk is through open foxtail pine forest. The forest floor is bare, save scattered individuals of a few species. One is the Sierra penstemon, a slightly spreading herb with a circular arrangement of skinny, tubular, purple flowers that are about 2 centimeters long. Another is Nuttall's sandwort, a straggly, mat-like plant with small, star-shaped, white flowers and needle-shaped leaves. The banks along small trickles and streams are densely covered with several mat-forming species, including carpet clover, with small white flowers, and primrose monkeyflower. Primrose monkeyflower has single, yellow, tubular flowers attached atop 2- to 4-inch stalks. It is always identifiable by its light green leaves pressed flat to the ground and long hairs that hold the morning dew and cause the plants to glow in the sun. Throughout the forest you will be greeted by small groups of dark-eyed juncos. These large sparrows, with dark heads and streaks of white on their tails, are the most common birds along the JMT. There are a few scattered campsites toward the northwestern end of Sandy Meadow, including, just as you leave the meadow, large campsites to the west, the direction of the old trail. You now climb slightly up another sandy shoulder, entering an open forest of foxtail pines and soon reach the apex of Mt. Young's shoulder [10,963' − 2.0/12.4]. When some small trickles of water are flowing, sandy patches here would make elegant campsites with the artistic pine trees, huge boulders, and a filtered view across to the Kaweah Peaks.

Shortly, you descend again and cross a small creek, beside which is one small tent site beneath lodgepole pines. As you descend a steeper, foxtail-pine-covered slope, you pass granite that is pinkish due to potassium feldspar, one of the minerals in granite. Here it is easily visible, as the granite has a greater percent of potassium feldspar and the individual rectangular crystals are large. Elsewhere, fractured boulders have greenish surfaces; this is the mineral epidote, which commonly fills small cracks in granite. Where the slope eases, you once again transition to lodgepole forest—the tree species each thrive in a slightly different environment—and turn west toward the Wallace Creek crossing. On the south bank are popular campsites and a bear box. Note that

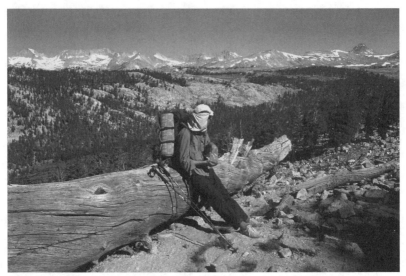

The Great Western Divide viewed on the descent beyond Bighorn Plateau

campfires are not permitted within 1200 feet of the bear box. You then cross Wallace Creek, which can be difficult early season, for although the rocks underfoot are small, it is a long crossing. You immediately reach the High Sierra Trail junction [10,405′ – 1.5/13.9], which goes west to the Giant Forest, while the JMT bends to the right.

You now climb up a steep, sandy slope with pennyroyal, Nuttall's sandwort, and more. At the summit, you enjoy a wonderful vista to the Kaweahs, cross a forested flat, and ford Wright Creek, possibly difficult in early season, as the water can be deep [10,700′ – 0.7/14.6]. There are good campsites just before this crossing and additional possibilities on the next stretch of trail as you parallel the creek eastward. For the next few miles, you cross many a sandy flat, often covered with low-growing lupines. Elsewhere, you skirt along the top of long meadows with small streams, tributaries of Wright Creek, many of which are filled with Bigelow's sneezeweed. A hardscrabble, sandy slope marks the remnants of an old moraine along the edge of the Wright Creek drainage. An additional ascent brings you to Bighorn Plateau [11,415′ – 1.9/16.5], named for sheep once seen in the area. Ironically, the plateau itself is lousy sheep habitat, and bighorn sheep tend to stick to cliffy areas where they can outmaneuver predators. Sandy, flat, unvegetated patches make for possible campsites with outstanding views, and the nearly round tarn just adds to the beauty. The vista of the northern Great Western Divide is especially fantastic. From south to north are Milestone Mountain, a narrow pinnacle; Midway Mountain, a not-too-inspiring peak; Table Mountain, with vertical sides and a flat top; and Thunder Mountain, a steep and imposing pyramid. But even if you don't spend a night here, plan ahead to spend some time, as the location is magical: Early in the morning, you'll likely hear packs of coyotes; a few hours later, you can watch the ravens sitting in the foxtail pine snags; American kestrels and other birds of prey will soar above you; and marmots will sun themselves on nearby boulders. In case the view isn't quite good enough, climb up Tawny Point, for the full panorama (see Appendix E), or wander westward to one of the shorter knobs overlooking the Kern drainage.

You now descend, skirting around the western side of Tawny Point, first across a barren landscape of sandy ground broken only by tufts of sedges, then onto exposed slopes dominated by foxtail pines, and finally through dry lodgepole forest. After some distance, you reach the Tyndall Frog Ponds, where there are large campsites, a bear box, warmish swimming, and beautiful views north to Diamond Mesa. Again, campfires are prohibited within 1200 feet of the camping area. Additional switchbacks bring you to a campsite and the first of three junctions you will encounter within the next half mile. This junction is with the trail that heads down Tyndall Creek. The Tyndall Creek ranger station is a little more than a half mile down this trail—much farther than is shown on many maps. Unless you wish to pay the ranger a visit, be sure to head right, turning uphill along the JMT, not down Tyndall Creek. (If you are using the USGS 7.5-minute maps, this will be counterintuitive, as they incorrectly show the Shepherd Pass Trail as branching off south of the Tyndall Creek Trail. Instead, the Shepherd Pass Trail junction is a short distance upstream—at 10,890 – 2.0/18.5.) In a few more steps, you reach the Tyndall Creek crossing, which, although short, can be formidable in early season because of the fast-flowing, freezing-cold water and rocky bottom. Just beyond the stream is the Tyndall Creek bear box and camping area. Please camp in the locations specified by the ranger and once again note that campfires are prohibited within 1200 feet of the crossing. You next reach a signed junction for the now unmaintained Lake South America Trail, taking you to the true headwaters of the Kern River, and a beautiful basin to explore if time permits [11,050' – 0.3/18.8].

Approximately following Tyndall Creek, you begin the final climb to Forester Pass. If, beyond one small stand of mixed lodgepole and foxtail pines, you turn around, you will get your last view of Mt. Whitney, the tall, flat-topped peak with large avalanche chutes on its northern

SEE MAPS 1–2

face. As you climb, you may find that the trail's exact location doesn't match your map, as it has been rerouted to minimize damage to the streamside vegetation. Indeed, you pass several small seeps with abundant mountaineer shooting stars, mountain monkeyflower, carpet clover, and more. Marmots are everywhere in this terrain, sunning themselves conspicuously atop the biggest boulders they can find. If you wish, you can make a side trip up Caltech Peak, to your left, which overlooks the Lake South America Basin and the Kings-Kern Divide. To do this, head west where the slope lessens and you can see large lakes to either side of the trail (see Appendix E).

You now begin a delightful walk up the broad, gentle valley. To the east, the steep faces of Junction Peak and Diamond Mesa are incongruous. The summits of these peaks were never glaciated, and the steep, smooth chutes on their western faces are all the result of avalanche activity. Only the lower reaches of the peaks bear signs of past glaciation: Note the boundary between "steep chute" and "nearly vertical wall," as this marks the height to which the valley was once filled with ice. For many miles, you wander through this sandy landscape, dotted by boulders and alpine tarns of all sizes, and with abundant fellfield species covering the ground. Three different species of buckwheat share this area: The yellow-flowered frosted buckwheat, a common species from the alpine down into montane forests, forms large mats and is easily identified by its small, fuzzy leaves and ball-like heads of minute yellow flowers that turn red as they go to seed. A white- to pink-flowered buckwheat with oval-shaped leaves, bearing such dense hairs that they appear nearly white is oval-leaved buckwheat. A second yellow-flowered species with spade-shaped leaves and long flower stalks lying horizontally on the ground is foxtail buckwheat, which you will not see again once you cross Forester Pass. Growing so close to the ground allows these plants to avoid persistent wind chill and to maintain leaf temperatures that are warmer than the surrounding air. Shortly, you cross the nascent Tyndall Creek for the last time [12,480' – 3.6/22.4].

After passing a few small, very exposed sandy patches that could hold a small tent, you begin the final switchbacking climb to the summit of Forester Pass. The first stretch is on talus, but shortly you reach the base of cliffs and admire the tenacity of both the alpine plants and the trail engineers. Growing on this near-vertical cliff face are club-moss ivesia, as always sticking out from cracks, and rockfringe, growing from the base of boulders and outcrops. You climb numerous exposed switchbacks, some of which are cut into the rock and others of which are built atop stone walls. It's not surprising that trail engineers had

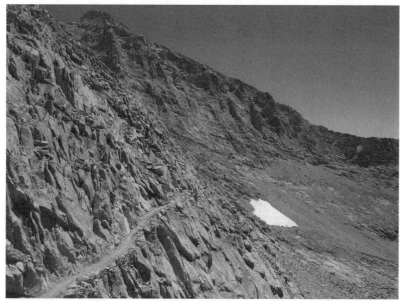

Trail to Forester Pass

initially planned to route the JMT elsewhere. A circuitous route was first constructed through Center Basin, to the northeast, then across Junction Pass, taking hikers east of the crest, and finally back across Shepherd Pass, to merge again with the current JMT route near the Tyndall Creek crossing. However, by 1931, the route over Forester Pass was discovered, scouted, and built, streamlining the route south to Whitney. In winter, however, skiers still use creative route-finding to successfully cross this divide. When you reach the summit, enjoy your last breathtaking and vast view of the Kern drainage: To the southwest are the dark, jagged summits of the Kaweahs, to their east is the long, straight fault scarp through which flows the Kern River, and straight ahead lies the magnificent rolling tundra landscape through which you have walked [13,100' – 0.8/23.2].

SEE MAP 2

SECTION 11.

Forester Pass to Glen Pass—Bubbs Creek Fork of the Kings River

Forester Pass is atop the Kings-Kern Divide, the border between the Kern River drainage that you have been in since Trail Crest and the Kings River drainage to the north. It is also the border between Kings Canyon and Sequoia national parks. Specifically, you are now in the Bubbs Creek drainage, the southernmost fork of the South Fork of the Kings. While the Kern River runs north-south, and your ascents and descents were relatively minor, the Kings River has many east-west-trending forks, resulting in one high pass after another. Looking north at this terrain, you can make out a jagged row of peaks in the distance, the Palisades, which lie just to the north of Mather Pass, many days' walk from here.

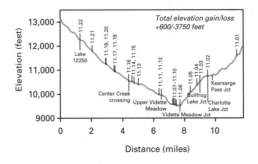

SEE MAP 2

Although sky pilot and club-moss ivesia were present on the pass, as you begin your descent down rocky switchbacks, you see very little growing. On the slope beneath Mt. Whitney, there were abundant plants at this elevation, but this is a north-facing slope, and snow may linger very late. Most species cannot grow during the brief snow-free weeks, and many others will emerge from rootstock only following the milder winters. Shortly, you find yourself descending a narrow spine, and your views of the Kings-Kern Divide and Mt. Stanford, the vertical face to the west, begin to open up. If you are lucky, you may see a golden eagle soaring high above these sharp summits. The sandy, flatter section of trail on which you are now walking sports Sierra cutleaf daisies, frosted buckwheat, and wax currant. Also present are pussytoes: Their long, skinny, dark green, and slightly succulent leaves hug the ground, and they have small balls of pink flowers on short stalks. You now descend switchbacks and shortly reach the outlet of Lake 12,250 (or Lake 12,090 on older maps) [12,250' – 1.3/1.3]. Barren and stark, there are some small tent and bivy sites in the talus to the east of the outlet. These have the potential for a beautiful sunset view of Junction Peak reflecting in the lake. You continue your descent through talus, passing more sky pilot and alpine gold. Enjoy them, for this is the last time the JMT is high enough that they will be common. These talus fields are also home to alpine chipmunks and pikas, small, round members of the rabbit

Location	Elevation	Distance from Previous Point	Cumulative Distance	UTM Coordinates
Forester Pass	13,100	—	0	11S 377385E 4061650N
Lake at 12,250 feet	12,250	1.3	1.3	11S 377826E 4062513N
Center Basin Creek crossing	10,540	3.1	4.4	11S 377503E 4065728N
Upper Vidette Meadow bear box	9945	2.1	6.5	11S 375571E 4068228N
Bubbs Creek junction	9515	1.2	7.7	11S 374004E 4068999N
Bullfrog Lake junction	10,515	1.3	9.0	11S 374109E 4069881N
Charlotte Lake junction	10,740	0.5	9.5	11S 373761E 4070152N
Kearsarge Pass junction	10,760	0.3	9.8	11S 373529E 4070466N
Glen Pass	11,960	2.0	11.8	11S 374134E 4072250N

SEE MAP 2

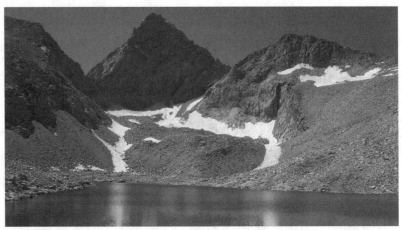

Lake 12,250 with Junction Peak in the background

family with adorable Mickey Mouse ears. When disturbed, these critters emit a two-noted *cheep-cheep*. Most impressively, this species does not hibernate in winter, but lives beneath talus piles, eating piles of hay it has prepared in summer.

At the base of the talus, you approach an alpine meadow and slab-strewn bench, the first in many miles. This landscape is the home of water pipets, spotted sandpipers, and gray-crowned rosy finches. Water pipets and spotted sandpipers are both especially common in Center Basin, to the east, with its expansive, wet, hummocky, alpine meadows. To your right is a large, steep-fronted pile of talus, a rock glacier. At this point in your journey, you have not yet passed by any of the Sierra's snow glaciers, but when you do, consider that all current glaciers in the Sierra Nevada formed during the Little Ice Age, a cold period that began 700 years ago. The much larger Pleistocene glaciers had completely disappeared in the interim. In contrast, the ice at the center of rock glaciers may be much older, possibly providing a longer climatic record for the Sierra—if only there were an easy way to core into it. As you pass through, you will see occasional sandy tent spots among meadows and slabs. If you wish to camp up in this alpine environment, please be sure to choose previously used locations to limit your impact on resources in this fragile area. Moving rocks exposes the roots of the small alpine plants, causing them to desiccate and likely die. You now descend a few more switchbacks, passing Sierra primrose, oval-leaved buckwheat, frosted buckwheat, mountain sorrel, and many other alpine species, before descending to another small meadow, and shortly reaching the first tree. From here on, the JMT will not take you

SEE MAP 2

so far above treeline, as the remaining passes are all 1000 feet lower than Forester Pass.

At the far western edge of this meadow is one small, exposed campsite (with magnificent views, of course), followed by a second one just below, in a clump of whitebark pines. You continue your descent, passing more meadows, creeks, and a few last piles of talus. West of the trail, you come upon a few sandy knobs, on which there are campsites nestled beneath whitebark pines. These, of course, come with spectacular views up and down Bubbs Creek. Just below, you cross some small streams. The ground is marshy and vegetation includes mountaineer shooting stars, primrose monkeyflower, and other species that you will see increasingly. One is little elephant's heads, which have elongate heads and small lavender flowers. If you look at an individual flower upside down, you can see its eponymous ears and trunk. Another is Lemmon's paintbrush, with tubular, beaked flowers just like the wavy-leaved paintbrush but with "brushes" that are a purple-magenta color.

Slowly, the scattered whitebark pines give way to a denser lodgepole forest. You pass the first forested campsites in many miles, and reach the Center Basin Creek crossing, a ford that can be high in early season [10,540' – 3.1/4.4]. A short distance later, you pass large campsites and a bear box. Just beyond, you pass a small cairn and a conspicuous line of rocks indicating the start of the trail—the only remaining marker for the Center Basin Trail junction. Before long, you again leave the lodgepole forest, now entering a landscape that, for large distances, is covered with downed tree limbs, evidence of past avalanches. Pioneer plants in this landscape include fireweed, a very tall species bearing clusters of quite large, four-petal, pink flowers that look similar to rockfringe, and low-growing willows. Due to this disturbance, your views are open; be sure to look up at the steep walls of East Vidette. In places, you come close to Bubbs Creek, where you can take a break beside the wonderful cascades and pools. In this vegetation, you may well spot American robins, a species of thrush with a burnt red belly. After a slightly steeper descent, you reach Upper Vidette Meadow, where there are bear boxes and good campsites both along the main creek and near the several tributaries you cross [9,945' – 2.1/6.5]. The trail continues through bare lodgepole forest. In places, the only plants growing here are species of rock cress, with small, white to purple, four-petal flowers on a tall stem. By midseason, most individual plants no longer have flowers and are instead decorated by long seedpods; species of rock cress are distinguished by the width of the pods and whether they are upright or drooping. Shortly, the trail emerges onto a

SEE MAP 2

steeper, open slope, before leveling out at Vidette Meadow. Here, there are large campsites, a bear box, and another excellent view of the east face of East Vidette, cut by steep avalanche chutes. Progressing ever northward, you again walk through barren stretches of forest, cross the outlet from Bullfrog Lake (a ford that can be a wade in early season) and reach the Bubbs Creek Trail junction [9515' – 1.2/7.7], where there are again large, shady campsites. Here, the Bubbs Creek Trail continues downstream to Roads End at Cedar Grove, while the JMT resumes its upward march.

Much of the next 1000-foot climb is through lodgepole forest, providing welcome shade. Twice you cross one of the two outlet streams descending from Bullfrog Lake. By each of them are small tent sites. In places, there is little groundcover and elsewhere there are thickets of sticky alpine currant, large ferns, and Bigelow's sneezeweed. Alongside the stream crossings is a community of plants that occurs at just about every stream crossing up to treeline. Three of these plants, all standing close to 2 feet tall, are swamp onion, great red paintbrush, and Kelley's tiger lily. Swamp onion has purple flowers and a pungent onion smell; great red paintbrush has large, bright red flowers and is the only Sierra paintbrush that prefers streams and seeps; Kelley's tiger lily sports large orange flowers with six reflexed petals. At long last, you reach the next junction, with the trail to Bullfrog Lake, the Kearsarge Lakes Basin, and, ultimately, to Kearsarge Pass [10,515' – 1.3/9.0]. There is a small tent site near the junction, but camping is prohibited at Bullfrog Lake and stock are prohibited on this trail. If you must exit to Independence to resupply, this is the shortest route to Kearsarge Pass.

After the brief flat, the climb resumes, this time up a short, steep slope with rocky footing. At the top, you cross an exposed knob with foxtail pines and briefly descend through whitebark and lodgepole pines. Shortly, you reach a large, sandy flat with the Charlotte Lake junction [10,760' – 0.5/9.5]. There is ample camping, a bear box, and a ranger station at the northeastern end of Charlotte Lake. You may also choose to detour to Charlotte Lake to climb Mt. Bago, which provides excellent views of the Kings-Kern and Great Western divides—views that are lacking from Glen Pass (see Appendix E.) Alternatively, heading east from this junction also takes you to Kearsarge Pass. A short distance up the JMT, you encounter one last junction toward Kearsarge Pass, which is used as an exit point by southbound hikers [10,760' – 0.3/9.8].

The trail now climbs up a dry, west-facing slope above Charlotte Lake. Pennyroyal, Fremont's groundsel, wavy-leaved paintbrush, frosted buckwheat, and Sierra primrose are among the many species

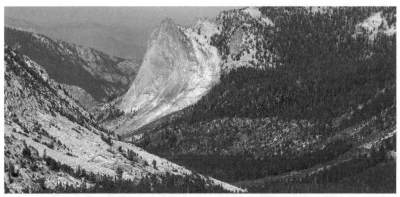

Charlotte Dome viewed from the traverse above Charlotte Lake

present. You will also see mountain pride penstemon, a low-growing shrub with serrate leaves and tubular magenta flowers, and western wallflower, a tall-stalked herb with a loose head of four-petal, yellow flowers. Where the trail bends eastward, stop and look back toward Charlotte Lake and extensive views to the west: Charlotte Dome is the steep, polished dome downstream. For a short stretch, you now enter sparse lodgepole forest, but then climb back into talus, passing a pothole lake with brilliant blue water. Behind the lake is a steep-fronted pile of talus, another rock glacier.

You ascend a few switchbacks and reach a second small lake. This one has small tent sites nestled among the whitebark pines on the southwest side of the lake. Skirting the lake along its western edge, you pass an area vegetated with red mountain heather and Sierra primroses growing among boulders. Begin your final climb to the pass, switchbacking up a dry, loose scree slope to Glen Pass. Up you go, past more Sierra primrose, pennyroyal, mountain sorrel, western wallflowers, wax currant, cliff bush, rockfringe, and a few alpine gold and sky pilots. Also growing here is shaggy hawkweed, which resembles a miniature yellow dandelion with leaves, covered with long, shaggy hairs. Granite gilia is a low-growing shrub with needle-like leaves and white-light pink, five-petal flowers whose bases form a tight cone and whose petal tips are more open. Finally, you reach the long, narrow summit of Glen Pass [11,960' – 2.0/11.8]. Your view south from Glen Pass is mostly blocked by the steep-walled cirque, out of which you have ascended. However, to the southwest, you can see the northern tip of the Great Western Divide: Pyramid-shaped Mt. Brewer is flanked by the unimpressive South Guard and notably steep North Guard.

SEE MAP 3

SECTION 10.

Glen Pass to
Pinchot Pass—Woods Creek Fork
of the Kings River

Now you turn around and look north toward the Rae Lakes, where you will head next. Like the Bubbs Creek drainage, Woods Creek is a tributary of the South Fork of the Kings River; their confluence is near Roads End. From an aerial perspective, your coming walk may appear to pass through barren country, but soon after you pass the first talus basin ahead, you will be walking through meadows and past lakes. You descend the switchbacks, the first few of which may hold snow all summer. As you descend, take note of the small and barely visible cushion plants. Where the grade lessens, club-moss ivesia appears in nearly every crack in the abundant slabs. And then you cross a small, flat basin with a collection of austere mountain tarns amongst the talus and slabs. A few minute sandy patches to your left may beckon to you as campsites. Alternatively, if you wish to detour to climb the Painted

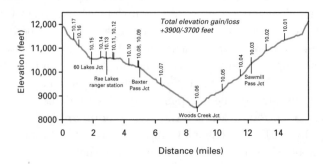

SEE MAP 3

Lady, which offers outstanding views of the Rae Lakes, it is on this flat that you leave the trail (see Appendix E). As you continue downward, keep your eyes open, as these next miles are where you are most likely to see Sierra Nevada bighorn sheep. You pass through sheep habitat several times on your journey, but the animals are both rare and difficult to spot—"boulders with legs," in the words of one researcher. However, for the last several years, a herd of rams has often been spotted here atop rocky knobs or in talus. Where you reach the first trees, knobs to the east of the trail provide small campsites with views downcanyon. You cross several small streams and descend through scattered tree cover to the shore of the upper Rae Lake and shortly reach the Sixty Lakes Basin Trail junction [10,545' – 1.9/1.9]. This exquisite subalpine basin is worth exploring if you have a few hours to spare, as the views of Mt. Clarence King are even more sublime, and the lakes are stunning. Scattered campsites exist west and northwest of the junction.

Your next many miles are through the Rae Lakes Basin, a flat walk through lush subalpine terrain, a scenic and highly used area with a well-earned reputation for bad mosquitoes. Be sure to read the campsite regulations that are posted at the Sixty Lakes Basin junction and accept that there are few camping options outside of the large camping areas beside bear boxes—you can expect company each night. Ford the connecting stream between the middle and upper Rae Lakes, and then proceed between the two on a narrow isthmus, where no camping is allowed. As you cross the isthmus, look at the views to the south and east—colorful metamorphic rock, especially on the face of the Painted Lady, decorate the head of the canyon. To the east, you see the blocky

Location	Elevation	Distance from Previous Point	Cumulative Distance	UTM Coordinates
Glen Pass	11,960	—	0	11S 374134E 4072250N
60 Lakes Basin junction	10,545	1.9	1.9	11S 374962E 4073715N
Rae Lakes ranger station	10,580	1.0	2.9	11S 375124E 4074637N
Baxter Pass junction	10,200	2.1	5.0	11S 374508E 4077248N
Woods Creek junction	8492	3.7	8.7	11S 371810E 4081629N
Sawmill Pass junction	10,345	3.5	12.2	11S 375312E 4084783N
Pinchot Pass	12,130	3.7	15.9	11S 374301E 4088514N

SEE MAP 3

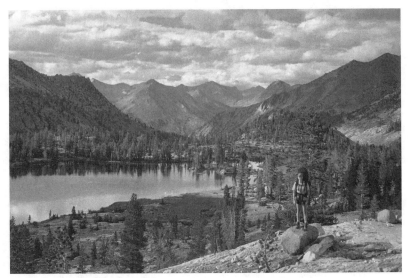

View north from the Rae Lakes

outline of the Sierra Crest near Dragon Peak. Your next camping option is near the south end of middle Rae Lake, where a sign points toward the lake's shore, to a large camping area with bear boxes.

As the trail veers south again, you pass one of the basin's many marshy meadows, and birds are abundant here. Yellow-rumped warblers, the all-yellow Wilson's warblers, and white-crowned sparrows are likely darting in an out of willows at the edge of meadows. Sitting atop whitebark pines are likely Clark's nutcrackers, a noisy and common relative of the jays. This light grey and black bird feeds on pine nuts and congregates from the upper elevation lodgepole forests to the timberline. More amazing is its natural history: It breeds in March in the Sierra, so unless you are on skis, you will never see the young. It sustains itself through the winter by eating from large stashes of whitebark pine nuts, buried on a diversity of slope aspects to ensure a continuous supply as the snow melts. You now traverse along the east side of the lakes, crossing many little flower-filled seeps and looking out across the lakes and westward to the steep peaks of the King Spur: Mt. Cotter and Mt. Clarence King. Wetter areas are covered with swamp onion, joined by great red paintbrush, Bigelow's sneezeweed, and the white Coulter's daisy, which has many exquisitely narrow ray petals. Also present is the Sierra rein orchid, bearing very small, white, orchid-shaped flowers on leafy stalks. As you traipse downcanyon, you next pass a sign marking the location of the Rae Lakes ranger station, a short

SEE MAP 3

distance east of the trail [10,580′ – 1.0/2.9]. At the lowest Rae Lake are another bear box and a large camping area among scattered whitebark pines.

You now pass Fin Dome, the prominent, steep, granite dome to the west, and resume your descent, in places through forest cover and elsewhere across dry flats. Although these openings appear grass-covered, they are inhabited by a group of related species, sedges, whose flowers are in small, dark heads. Sometimes individual plants appear as circles, where they have grown outward over many years. A characteristic group of species is found on these flats: Parish's yampah is a member of the carrot family, with three linear leaf-lobes and a broad head of minute white flowers. Also abundant in these flats are two species of pussytoes, which form extensive mats and have small, elongate, and quite fuzzy leaves and flowers that resemble small tufts of fuzz. Rosy pussytoes flowers have a pinkish tinge, while others, such as flat-top pussytoes, are white. Pussypaws and Sierra penstemon may also be present. Your descent levels out at the edge of Arrowhead Lake. At this lake, ringed by a large meadow and reeds, there are campsites both under lodgepole forest near a bear box and on more exposed slabs a bit north. The sunset and sunrise reflections of Fin Dome are phenomenal both here and at Dollar Lake, a short distance downstream—take your pick. To reach Dollar Lake, proceed around the marshy shore of Arrowhead Lake, pass a small and colorful meadow, cross the outlet on a small bridge, and proceed downstream. As you approach Dollar Lake, you pass a cliff face, below which grow pink heuchera, cliff bush, and the bright red-orange crimson columbine, whose flowers point upright and have five long spurs that dangle behind. At the northwest corner of the lake are campsites on open, sandy patches among granite slabs. From here departs the Baxter Pass Trail, an unmaintained and disappearing trail headed eastward [10,200′ – 2.1/5.0].

The terrain now becomes rockier and drier. You emerge onto dark-colored granitic slabs in a stark landscape of scattered foxtail pines, which have replaced lodgepole pines. This is the last time you will see a large stand of this southern Sierra species. You descend through this open landscape for some time. One of the few species common alongside outcropping rock is Sierra stonecrop, a succulent with small, yellow, star-like flowers. Lower down, where you re-enter forest cover, is a burgundy-colored succulent, rosy sedum, which thrives in rocky seeps and on wetter forest floor. You cross a small tributary, and then where the trail trends left, away from the water, you encounter a campsite; the better camping option is downstream of the trail. Farther along, you

SEE MAP 3

pass a large, marshy meadow filled with wildflowers. By late season, three species of gentian will be blooming here: the stalkless, white alpine gentian; Sierra gentian, with a single, narrow, tubular purple flower on a 4-inch stalk; and the periwinkle-colored perennial swertia, with numerous flowers on an 8-inch stalk. By August, the alpine gentian and Sierra gentian are widespread meadow constituents throughout the Sierra, while perennial swertia is rare to the north.

You cross the marsh's channel on a small bridge and continue downstream, sometimes in forest, sometimes on dry knobs, eventually fording a stream draining lakes on the northern tip of the King Spur; the water can be deep in early season. Increasingly, you cross long sections with dry, open knobs, on which grow small sedge meadows as well as mountain pride penstemon, Nuttall's sandwort, and wavy-leaved paintbrush. The aromatic shrub mountain sagebrush, with grey-green, three-lobed leaves, may also be present. Lower still, you re-enter lodgepole forest, and as you approach the valley bottom, a section of cobble-covered forest floor provides evidence of past flood events. Shortly, to the right of the trail, you reach a large camping area and two bear boxes beneath Jeffrey pines, red firs, and a few lodgepole pines. To the south are additional campsites near a juniper-covered knob. Red fir, with deep red bark and short, individually attached needles, grows only below 9000 feet, and this forest is the first time you have seen it. However, it will become common as you reach the lower-elevation forests to the north. Western juniper is a conifer, but its needles are so reduced that they appear as small scales and its cones as berries. These trees always stand alone and are most artistic with their curved branches and shaggy red bark. The ever-squawking Steller's jays, dark blue birds with a black crest, will be hopping around camp in search of an untended snack. Just beyond the camping area, you cross roaring Woods Creek on an imposing, narrow, and very bouncy suspension bridge, the "Golden Gate of the Sierra," completed in 1988 and not subject to washouts like its predecessor. (One person at a time, please!) The trail now trends slightly west to the junction with the Woods Creek Trail [8,492' – 3.7/8.7], which goes south down Woods Creek, past Paradise Valley, to Cedar Grove.

Back up again. Make sure you get an early start, as the first part of this climb provides no shade. You ascend a manzanita-covered slope dotted with Jeffrey pines and western juniper. If you turn around, you have a good view of the towering walls around you—Castle Domes to the north, and the King Spur to the south. To your side is the stream, cascading down smooth slabs. As you ascend further, on the south side

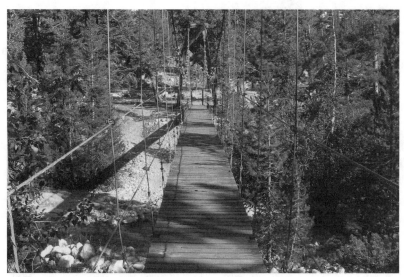

Woods Creek bridge

of the creek, is a well-delineated moraine, the piles of material pushed to the side by a glacier that once flowed down this canyon. As you climb, you pass several streams, and although these will all be wades in early season, the crossings are flat with good foot purchase on small- to medium-sized rocks. Only the White Fork tributary, with its rockier substrate, is likely to be difficult. You approach the end of the Jeffrey pines and western junipers when you reach a bench with a collection of campsites that are mostly quite small. Just steps farther along are your very last foxtail pines—admire them one last time. You continue fol- lowing the creek's north shore, with eye-catching views into the small stream gorge and, at one point, some small cascades. Up ahead looms a long talus field that is, from a distance, dotted by willows and scrubby quaking aspen, with bright white bark and slightly pointed leaves. As you walk through it, the smaller herbs become apparent: wavy-leaved paintbrush, scarlet penstemon, pennyroyal, and Sierra angelica, sport-ing an enormous spherical head of miniature white flowers on a tall stalk. Above the talus field, you enter lodgepole forest and immedi-ately pass a good campsite and cross a side creek. Drier sections of for-est floor are covered in sticky alpine currant, but on a wetter slope, Bigelow's sneezeweed and Kelley's tiger lily appear. Joining them is ranger's buttons, a species that superficially resembles Sierra angelica, except it bears many tight "buttons" of white flowers, each on their own stalk. The plant with the largest, ovate leaves and possibly a long

SEE MAP 3

stem of white flowers, is the corn lily. Early in the season, these look like ears of corn, but by summer they are tall and straggly. Out of forest cover again, you ascend a few more dry switchbacks among multicolored slabs and reach the junction for the Sawmill Pass Trail [10,345′ − 3.5/12.2]; a few exposed campsites lie on the bench just east of this junction, across the multistranded creek. The Kings Canyon side of this trail is now being maintained after a long hiatus.

The trail proceeds upward, through whitebark and lodgepole forest, across metamorphic slabs and sandy patches, and past dry sedge meadows. The latter are often dotted with small yellow flowers resembling dandelions: alpineflames. Elsewhere, you may have seen the superficially similar short-beaked agoseris, but this species lacks the central disc seen in the alpineflames, such that the multi-length ray petals merge to a single point. When you skirt the edge of a small lake, you can find camping on small knobs east of the trail, the last large ones until you are across Pinchot Pass. Beyond these lakes, the trail heads west and out of the drainage, to avoid damaging the delicate meadow vegetation. You are instead traversing sparsely forested sandy flats and, up higher, talus and rocky outcrops. The sandy flats often contain Muir's ivesia, one of the few plants to bear his name. These are small yellow flowers on long stalks with dense stalks of minute, fuzzy leaves that resemble a mouse's tail. As you approach the final meadows below Pinchot Pass, look down on an enchanting series of ponds and lakes—if you don't have time for a break now, come back just to visit them someday. Alternately, Crater Mountain, to the west, has an amazing vista south to the King Spur, if you have half a day to spare (see Appendix E). The last wet areas before you reach the switchbacks contain abundant mountaineer shooting stars and rosy sedum. And as your puff your way to the summit, scan the surrounding red metamorphic mountains for bighorn sheep. Finally, you reach the pass and, turning around, you can look back toward Woods Creek one last time [12,130′ − 3.7/15.9].

SEE MAPS 3–4

SECTION 9.

Pinchot Pass to Mather Pass— South Fork of the Kings River

The much-fractured metamorphic rock that composed Pinchot Pass leads to peaks that are piles of loose scree. However, this rock decomposes to form a fertile, moist soil in which plants thrive. Just below the pass, thriving in these wet conditions, is the delightful Eschscholtz' buttercup, identified by its deeply lobed leaves. As you descend toward Lake Marjorie, you find yourself almost constantly surrounded by meadows with beautiful, flower-lined seeps. Small, sandy flats that are covered with masses of short, red, straggly stems, the remains of early-blooming bud saxifrage. Wet meadows are covered with primrose monkeyflower, Sierra penstemon, little elephant's head, and alpine aster, a light purple daisy, always with a single head, whose petals are incurved where they attach to the central disc. On moist slopes, you will see bush cinquefoil, shrubs covered with bright yellow flowers, each of whose five petals approximate the shape of a rose petal.

As you approach Lake Marjorie, the first exposed, sandy campsites are west of the trail. The JMT traces Lake Marjorie's eastern shore,

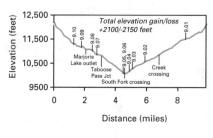

reaching the first whitebark pine krumholz. You'll find additional small tent sites tucked away in sandy patches beneath these stunted trees, both near Lake Marjorie's outlet and downstream near the first larger stream crossing [11,055' – 2.1/2.1]. This outlet and those downstream are all easily crossed, mostly on large blocks of rock. Along the way, be sure to stop and look north to Mather Pass: The impressively steep peak just north of the South Fork of the Kings is Mt. Ruskin. As you descend, you will pass several tarns. Campsites exist on slightly forested knobs near most of these. The Bench Lake ranger station is located on the northeast shore of the lake you reach just before the Bench Lake Trail junction. Note that this ranger station is not always occupied. If you have extra energy to walk another 2 miles, Bench Lake, perched high above the South Fork of the Kings River, has beautiful campsites along its northeastern shore, sporting justifiably famous sunrise reflections of Arrow Peak. Just beyond this junction, ford the creek draining from Pinchot Pass, step across a small trickle, and reach the junction with the Taboose Pass Trail [10,780' – 1.0/3.1].

You now begin a steep descent down a dry, south-facing slope beneath scattered lodgepole pines. Nuttall's sandwort and rock cress are two of the only species you'll find here. At the bottom, you ford a small creek and shortly reach the main South Fork of the Kings crossing [10,040' – 1.5/4.6], which can be quite difficult. In early season, you will want to wade across where the river splits around an islet downstream, and later in the season, you can hop across rocks a bit upstream. Some campsites near this crossing may be closed for restoration, but options abound.

Location	Elevation	Distance from Previous Point	Cumulative Distance	UTM Coordinates
Pinchot Pass	12,130	—	0	11S 374301E 4088514N
Crossing below Lake Marjorie	11,055	2.1	2.1	11S 372474E 4090150N
Taboose Pass junction	10,780	1.0	3.1	11S 371999E 4091458N
Main South Fork Kings crossing	10,040	1.5	4.6	11S 371517E 4092357N
South Fork Kings crossing at base of Upper Basin	10,860	2.2	6.8	11S 370783E 4095789N
Mather Pass	12,100	3.0	9.8	11S 370227E 4099161N

SEE MAP 4

You now begin the 2000-foot climb to the summit of Mather Pass, which is quite manageable compared to the climbs you've done up the last several passes. A short distance upstream, an old (although not quite vanished) trail descends the South Fork of the Kings, climbs over Cartridge Pass, and passes through Lakes Basin and down Cartridge Creek. This is the route the JMT followed temporarily while the trails up the Golden Staircase and Mather Pass were being built. Some distance farther upstream, near some good campsites, a rock cairn marks where an old trail, whose route you can still follow, climbs to Taboose Pass. Now you are in a lodgepole forest, and many sections have enough moisture for denser than usual understory vegetation, including corn lilies and mountaineer shooting stars. The JMT emerges from the forest and enters dry meadows, mostly dominated by sedges. Here there are abundant alpineflames, short-beaked agoseris, Parish's yampah, and pussytoes. The low-growing, sprawling dwarf bilberry, a type of blueberry with small, ovate leaves and bell-shaped flowers, is common where the ground is slightly moister. Unfortunately, it rarely bares fruit. Along this section, no campsites are obvious from the trail, but snooping eastward, in the direction of the river, yields some possibilities. Forest cover all but disappears by the time you next ford the river, still the South Fork of the Kings [10,860' – 2.2/6.8].

As you continue your climb, stop and admire the landscape. To the west are steep, glaciated, granite peaks, and to the east are craggy, colorful, metamorphic ones. For the next many miles, you are close to the contact between the older metamorphic rocks and the younger granitic ones. The precursors to these metamorphic rocks formed in their current location: seafloor-deposited sediments that were later compressed and twisted. Such material, termed "roof pendants," once overlay the granite through much of the Sierra, but it was eroded across much of the range as the granite core was uplifted, first about 50 million years ago, and more rapidly in the last 3 million to 5 million years. Cardinal Mountain, a massive red peak with a white tip, sticks out to the southeast: The red material was once sand and silt, while the white is marble, the remains of ocean critters deposited in a shallow reef environment. Meanwhile, to the west, you see a granite arête, Saddlehorn, and other steep walls to the north of Mt. Ruskin.

You continue up a gentle slope, crossing a few small tributaries en route, and find yourself in lake-dotted Upper Basin, another of the Sierra's treasures. These tarns, set in a bare, sandy landscape are incredibly enticing. Although no established campsites are visible from the trail, you can wander toward any of the tarns and may pitch your

SEE MAP 4

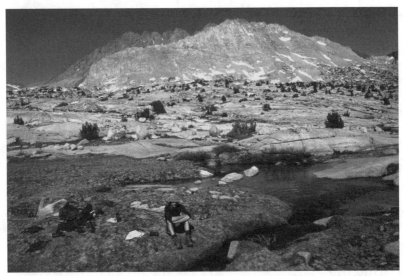

A lazy afternoon in Upper Basin with Mather Pass visible to the far left

tent on flat, sandy, unvegetated patches. You can easily spend hours sitting along their banks (sometimes on nearly bare sand, other times on polished slabs), and stare at the collection of insects and perhaps small tadpoles racing about. Or, if you wish to take a layover day in the vicinity, Split Mountain, the southernmost of the Palisade area four-teeners is a straightforward, if long, climb (see Appendix E). Along the sandy stretches, Muir's ivesia, frosted buckwheat, Sierra penstemon, pussypaws, and Nuttall's sandwort are common species. Joining them is the alpine paintbrush, not as dazzling and bright as the other species, but still elegantly colored. Growing just a few inches off the ground, the characteristic tubular flowers range from green to white to light pink, and the upper leaves sport a dainty white or pink edge. In wetter flats, you see little elephant's heads and alpine aster. There are also the diminutive arctic willows crawling along the ground, most easily iden-tifiable if covered by the white fuzz that accompanies their flowers. At the head of Upper Basin, you curve west and then ascend switchbacks to the summit of Mather Pass, named for Stephen Mather, the first head of the National Park Service [12,000' – 3.0/9.8].

SEE MAP 4

SECTION 8.

Mather Pass to Muir Pass—
Middle Fork of the Kings River

O n the summit of Mather Pass, you leave behind the many tributaries of the South Fork of the Kings River and enter the Middle Fork of the Kings watershed. While the South Fork drainages all converge near Cedar Grove, which is easily accessible by car, the Middle Fork drains down to Tehipite Valley, a long hike from anywhere, and then into an 8000-foot deep, trail-less gorge. Looking north from Mather Pass, you see the full length of the North and Middle Palisade peaks: Within view are six points that extend above the 14,000-foot mark. Ahead of you is a giant pile of granitic talus, so remarkably different from the meadows and streams on the north side of Pinchot Pass. You descend this barren country, seeing few species besides club-moss ivesia and Sierra primrose, the latter of which will become much more rare as you continue north. Lower, the trail turns north, the talus finally begins to diminish, and you

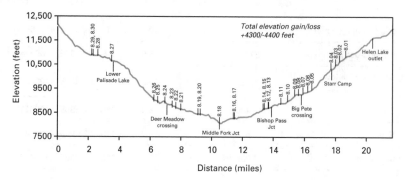

descend on small meadows toward the Palisade Lakes, all the while star-ing at the sharp-toothed Middle Palisade group. Shortly after the trail curves west to circle around the upper Palisade Lake, you pass the first stunted whitebark pines on small, sandy shelves. Some of these shelves hold view-rich campsites. Along this traverse, you ford an occasional stream, a few of which require a brief wade in early season. As you walk along, enjoy the view: the steep granite walls to the south, the jagged Palisades to the north, and the open valley ahead to the west. At the west end of the lower Palisade Lake [10,615' – 3.6/3.6], on slabs to the north of the trail, is one last, large campsite. It is sandy and barren, but has your last chance for these views before descending the Golden Staircase.

West of the Palisade Lakes, you continue for a short distance through pretty alpine meadows, fording a couple of tributaries. Alpine aster, dwarf bilberry, and alpine gentian are all present in the meadows. Mountain pride penstemon grows at the base of the adjoining rocks. Suddenly, the valley floor drops out beneath you and you can look nearly 1500 feet down to Deer Meadow. This, the Golden Staircase, was the last section of the JMT to be constructed and was completed in 1938. Impressively built walls form the foundation for the approximately 50 switchbacks that make for a steep climb down a much steeper head-wall. As you pound down the trail, look south to tumbling Palisade Creek, taking the direct route to Deer Meadow, and west to Devils

Location	Elevation	Distance from Previous Point	Cumulative Distance	UTM Coordinates
Mather Pass	12,100	—	0	11S 370227E 4099161N
Lower Palisade Lake outlet	10,615	3.6	3.6	11S 367705E 4102392N
Deer Meadow creek crossing	8830	3.5	7.1	11S 364338E 4101912N
Middle Fork junction	8070	3.4	10.5	11S 359647E 4101681N
Bishop Pass junction	8720	3.4	13.9	11S 358398E 4106234N
Big Pete Meadow creek crossing	9245	1.9	15.8	11S 357303E 4108387N
Starr Camp	10,480	2.3	18.1	11S 354585E 4108611N
Helen Lake outlet	11,615	2.3	20.4	11S 352659E 4109140N
Muir Pass	11,980	1.3	21.7	11S 351636E 4108416N

SEE MAP 4

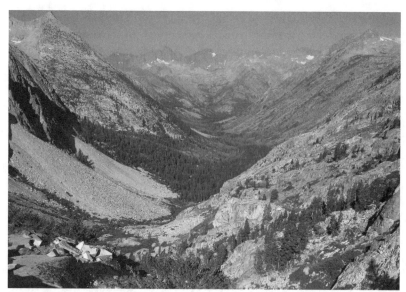

Palisade Creek and the Black Divide viewed from the top of the Golden Staircase

Crags, the dark, jagged mass of pinnacles at the southern end of the Black Divide. As always, what appeared from a distance to be barren rock is alive with flowers. The dry sections boast the ever more familiar wavy-leaved paintbrush, scarlet penstemon, pennyroyal, and shaggy hawkweed. As you drop lower, western eupatorium, a late-blooming species with a collection of light lavender heads lacking obvious petals, is added to the list. In the wetter sections, you will see swamp onion, Kelly's tiger lily, Sierra rein orchid, and great red paintbrush. Another wet-site species is the alpine goldenrod, with short, yellow, ray petals that look dwarfed relative to the size of the orange-yellow disc. Small-leaved cream bush, cliff bush, and pink heuchera emerge from cracks. Joining them is dense-flowered spiraea, another shrub whose clusters of bright rose-pink flowers are likely to catch your attention.

Finally, at the base of this long descent, you enter increasingly dense lodgepole forest and find several camping opportunities. You next cross the many forks of Glacier Creek, draining one of the basins at the foot of the 14,000-foot northern Palisade Peaks. You also pass through an often marshy section of trail and reach Deer Meadow, a lodgepole forest. Heading south from the trail, you find a couple of shaded campsites. Just beyond Deer Meadow, cross a stream draining Palisade Basin [8830' – 3.5/7.1].

Shortly, the lodgepole forest disappears and burnt snags and fallen logs suddenly surround you. Indeed, much of the next 3 miles was affected by the 2002 lightening-started Palisade Fire. Although there is now less forest, the herbaceous cover is lush and diverse. The trail is often indistinct as its passes through meadows, and there are downed trees from winter, making travel a bit slow in places. There are also far fewer camping opportunities than there were in the past, and as the vegetation changes during the next many years, the location of campsites will change. Currently, the best opportunities are in undisturbed stands of trees near the river or sandy shelves under Jeffrey pines to the north of the trail.

Toward the canyon bottom, the grade increases, and instead of burnt logs, you find yourself in a landscape of dense aspen scrub and manzanita. You suddenly emerge onto more open slabs dotted with towering Jeffrey pines and steep canyon walls in every direction. Just before you reach the low point, note on your left the remains of a bridge that once crossed Palisade Creek. Today, the junction with the Middle Fork of the Kings Trail is a short distance downstream [8070' – 3.4/10.5], and is signed. But unfortunately, the lack of a bridge makes it very difficult and dangerous to access during high water. It is here that the previously described route down Cartridge Creek rejoins the JMT. At this junction, there are several campsite present beneath the tall Jeffrey pines.

You have just descended 4000 feet from the summit of Mather Pass and immediately begin the 4000-foot climb to the top of Muir Pass, the last of the high passes along the JMT. For the first many miles, you climb up through Le Conte Canyon, a narrow valley with steep avalanche-prone sides. You will quickly note that there are few campsites that are 100 feet from the trail and/or water. Remember that the Kings Canyon regulations do allow you to camp in established sites 25 feet from trail/water, but you are not allowed to disturb the vegetation to create new campsites, even if they would place you a bit farther from the trail. Shortly, you reach Grouse Meadow, a long, skinny meadow with outstanding views of the canyon and with one of the largest blueberry patches in the Sierra. Unlike the dwarf bilberry, the western blueberries grow knee high and can have sufficient small blueberries for a quick snack. You will find several campsites along the length of the meadow. Farther upstream, you pass through sections of dry forest, mostly lodgepole, but with a few red fir present. The fir trees immediately stand out, for their quite short needles are attached singly to branches, and the bark of the adult trees is a rich red. In between areas of forest cover, you are walking across dry, open slopes, often the result of frequent avalanches or rockslides that prevent a conifer forest from establishing. As along Bubbs Creek, slopes covered by downslope-oriented tree trunks and vegetated by scrubby aspens are indicative of avalanche activity. In some open sections, you will note a mixture of two different manzanitas: One, pinemat manzanita, creeps along the ground, often under scattered tree cover, while the other, greenleaf manzanita, grows as a taller bush and has sticky glands on its leaf stalks. Both have scaly red bark, characteristic of all manzanita species. Several miles beyond Grouse Meadow, you enter some flatter stretches of forest (where you find the next campsites), shortly cross the turbulent Dusy Branch on a footbridge, and immediately pass additional campsites. In a few more steps, you reach the junction with the Bishop Pass Trail [8720' – 3.4/13.9], leading up into Dusy Basin and over Bishop Pass, the easiest access route to the town of Bishop.

Just thereafter, the JMT reaches the spur trail to the Le Conte Canyon ranger station. The trail now climbs more gradually and walking is pleasant on the soft forest floor. Before long, you come to Little Pete Meadow, which is, contrary to its name, large. A stream meanders through here. Also visible are oxbow lakes, which formed when the stream changed its course. To the edge are dense stands of corn lilies, a few of which will have many-branched heads of white flowers, but most senesce without flowering. There are a few campsites along the meadow's perimeter. Beyond the meadow, the trail briefly emerges from the forest, and you climb a sandy slope dotted with western junipers. There are phenomenal views westward to the steep face of Languille Peak. There is one small campsite here. You continue your gradual upward march through lodgepole forest, approaching Big Pete Meadow, which is mostly overgrown and can be difficult to spot from the trail. However, near a slight knob, an obvious spur trail does lead west to the river bank and campsites. Just thereafter, the trail bends west, passes additional small campsites, and crosses a multibranched side stream on logs [9245' – 1.9/15.8].

After the creek crossing, you continue along the forest trail, passing several more campsites. The trail then abruptly leaves the stream course (and forest cover), and you begin the long climb toward Muir Pass. The trail is now rocky underfoot, and you climb up dry slopes dominated by manzanita and chinquapin. To navigate through one section, the trail had to be blasted out of the canyon's sheer granite wall, and if you read Joseph N. Le Conte's account of the first descent through here, crisscrossing the valley multiple times to navigate around the

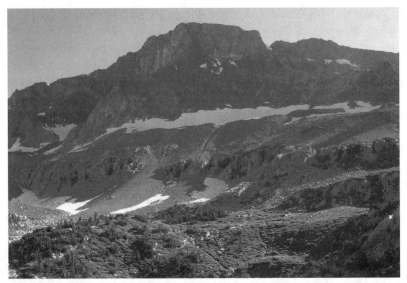

The Black Giant viewed from just beyond Starrs Camp

cliffs, you'll be glad for the work of dynamite. You climb high above the deep river gorge. Only near the top is the river again beside you, cascading down a steep granite slab. Here, you finally have scattered tree cover, and fireweed and large ferns grow where seeps and shade increase soil moisture. As the grade eases, look to your left: Here is a large flat of young lodgepole pines, a location long-ago named Starrs Camp [10,480′ – 2.3/18.1]. If you leave the trail here, you will find abundant camping opportunities in the direction of the creek, positioned at the top of the steep drop into Le Conte Canyon.

The trail now bends northward, passes a large, marshy meadow, and continues upward, switchbacking up a steeper slope and crossing a creek several times. Trickles of water abound and the vegetation is lush, with mountaineer shooting stars, red heather, and spreading carpets of Sierra arnica all making appearances. These large, yellow flowers, related to sunflowers, appear sporadically in open lodgepole forests. Clark's nutcrackers will be hopping among the treetops. Meanwhile, the east face of the Black Giant looms above; note how the peak's character changes at the contact between metamorphic and granitic rocks. The dark rock, part of the Goddard Terrane, is one of the largest masses of metamorphic rock in the Sierra. The action of plate tectonics smashed material into the continent between 150 million and 250 million years ago, leading to large volcanic eruptions. The subsequent tectonic action that created the Sierra Nevada's granite caused

SEE MAP 5

the volcanic rock to be metamorphosed, creating the dark rock you will see to the south of the trail for the next many miles. As you climb, a few large campsites present themselves under open stands of tall lodgepole pines. Near the 10,800-foot mark, you reach the next lake basin. Good campsites with stunning views lie among the stunted trees on the knob to the east of its outlet. For more than 10 miles, there are now few camping opportunities, so it is inadvisable to continue upward if the day is waning, especially if you have a large group. As you circumnavigate the unnamed lake, you ford a series of inlet streams—possible wades in early season. Climb ever onward, and note occasional granitic knobs sporting stunted whitebark pines. A small party may find camping opportunities on some of these knobs. A bit higher, the trail crosses onto metamorphic rock, and the knobs that emerge from the landscape become rockier and less hospitable for camping.

Leaving the last krumholz behind, you shortly reach a small, unnamed lake and follow the trail through a meadow filled with dense patches of mountaineer shooting stars interspersed with cobble-paved waterways. Above, the infant Middle Fork of the Kings River is confined to an enticing little gorge, paved with dark rock. The trail climbs to its right, and tall rock faces extend upward from the trail. Flowers, including mountain monkeyflower, primrose monkeyflower, and rockfringe, appreciate the abundant moisture and color their base. For stretches, the creek flows over the trail, but the water is minimal and doesn't impede your progress. Suddenly, the slope once again eases as you reach the outlet of Helen Lake, named for one of John Muir's daughters [11,615′ – 2.3/20.4]. As you encircle the lake, you'll enjoy its brilliant blue waters and the surrounding colorful glaciated slabs, for here the trail passes near the contact between metamorphic and granitic rocks. To the southeast lies the Black Giant, the northern end of the Black Divide and an easy peak with an excellent vista if you have half a day to spare (see Appendix E). You ascend the final switchbacks (rocky and sandy during dry summers) to Muir Pass, much of the time across a well-trodden path in the snow. Luckily, the grade is neither too steep nor too long, and shortly you reach Muir Pass [11,980′ – 1.3/21.7], where there is a stone hut intended to provide emergency shelter from storms. Camping in the area is prohibited because of human-waste problems. A marmot is always on guard at the hut—keep your eyes on your food at all times.

SEE MAP 5

SECTION 7.

Muir Pass to Selden Pass—South Fork of the San Joaquin River

A s you cross Muir Pass, you are entering the San Joaquin River drainage. With the exception of the 5 miles in the Rush Creek drainage, all the land you now traverse drains into the San Francisco Bay. In contrast, in the southern section that you just completed, water reaches the ocean only in wet years—mind-boggling when you consider the vast quantities of snow that bury this country each winter. The water from the Kern and Kings drainages once flowed into Tulare Lake, a vast wetland in the southern San Joaquin Valley, but today *all* of the water is diverted for irrigation and the Tulare lakebed is agricultural land.

Your next 5 miles will be spent tromping through undeniably spectacular Evolution Basin—make sure you have many hours to wander through it and to sit and absorb the scenery. This basin is also steeped

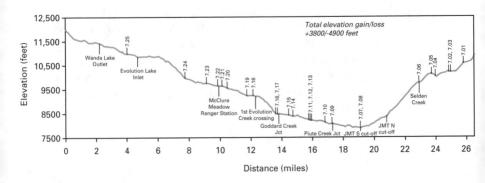

SEE MAP 5

in JMT history: In July 1895, Theodore Solomons, the visionary of the JMT, named the first six peaks of the Evolution Range after the most prominent figures in the new field of evolutionary biology: Darwin, Fiske, Haeckel, Huxley, Spencer, and Wallace, along with Evolution Lake. Although Solomons had first alighted on the idea of the JMT a decade earlier, it was on trips in 1895 and 1896 that he fleshed out his idea, in part while soaking up the landscape of Evolution Basin. His goal was to find a route between Yosemite and the South Fork of the Kings that stayed close to the crest and was passable by stock. During these summers, he traveled south from Yosemite to this region, but his parties then descended to the Middle Fork of the Kings by other routes. Unfortunately for them, then unnamed Muir Pass was, in both years, buried beneath an enormous snow bank, forcing them to search farther west for alternatives. Finally, in 1907 a US Geological Survey party crossed Muir Pass, and the following year, Joseph N. Le Conte used the pass as he continued scouting a route for the eventual JMT to the south. Climbing Solomons's namesake (Mt. Solomons), gives you a glimpse into the Ionian Basin, mostly composed of metamorphic rock and filled with crystal clear aqua lakes (see Appendix E).

Location	Elevation	Distance from Previous Point	Cumulative Distance	UTM Coordinates
Muir Pass	11,980	—	0	11S 351636E 4108416N
Wanda Lake outlet	11,420	2.2	2.2	11S 349266E 4110347N
Evolution Lake inlet	10,852	2.5	4.7	11S 349861E 4113857N
McClure Meadow ranger station	9640	5.2	9.9	11S 345384E 4116969N
Wade across Evolution Creek	9200	2.4	12.3	11S 341941E 4117861N
Goddard Creek junction	8480	1.5	13.8	11S 340782E 4117608N
Piute Creek junction	8050	3.5	17.3	11S 337415E 4121216N
JMT southern cutoff	7880	1.8	19.1	11S 334959E 4121342N
JMT northern cutoff	8400	1.7	20.8	11S 334054E 4123186N
Senger Creek crossing	9740	2.1	22.9	11S 334734E 4124423N
Selden Pass	10,890	3.6	26.5	11S 334070E 4128460N

SEE MAP 5

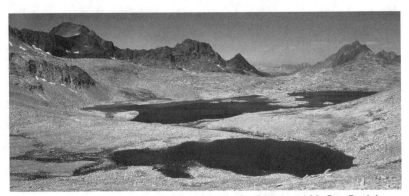

The upper lakes in Evolution Basin with Mt. Goddard and McGee Peak in the background

Descending from Muir Pass, you encircle Lake McDermand and shortly reach Wanda Lake's grassy east shore. This beautiful body of water is named for John Muir's other daughter. To the southwest rises the dark pyramidal mass of Mt. Goddard, the tallest of the peaks in the Ionian Basin, but the JMT itself is now back on granite slabs. You soon cross the multibranched outlet of Wanda Lake [11,420' – 2.2/2.2]. As you descend, stop and admire the many glacial features that surround you. During the last ice age, Evolution Basin was scoured clean, and the abundant glacial erratics scattered across the landscape attest to the glaciers' presence. Since then, little soil has formed, and the smooth granite slabs still dominate the landscape. Meanwhile, the upper sections of the highest peaks, Mt. Darwin and Mt. Mendel, were untouched by glaciers. Their summit regions are broad plateaus, the remnants of a long ago gentle Sierra landscape, which existed before a combination of uplift and river erosion, followed by glacial activity, created today's landforms. Beyond a pair of unnamed lakes, you begin a descending traverse high above the western shore of stunning Sapphire Lake. To the east is Mt. Spencer, an unremarkable peak from this angle, but one with a steep northern face, a fantastic view, and an easy ascent from the southwest (see Appendix E). You can descend straight to Sapphire Lake, but it is easier to continue along the JMT to its outlet and then backtrack along its eastern shore. There are also a few small campsites among the whitebark pines at the southern end of the lake.

You continue down a gentle slope, passing sandy stretches dotted with small alpine plants, meadows filled with a more vivid selection of flowers, and, to the east, a series of small lakes. The sandy flats often contain Muir's ivesia and alpine paintbrush. Meanwhile, Lemmon's

SEE MAPS 5–6

paintbrush, with the magenta flowers, grows in the wetter meadows you pass. Here you are also in the habitat of gray-crowned rosy finches. Shortly, you reach Evolution Lake's inlet, crossed on a series of large, granite blocks [10,852' – 2.5/4.7]. Skirt around the eastern shore of Evolution Lake, on a route constructed in the early 1990s to avoid the lake's sensitive shoreline. You are now passing beneath the massive wall of scalloped ridges and avalanche gullies descending from Mt. Mendel. Note where these giant slides are truncated, indicating the depth of ice during previous glacial periods. Within a short distance, you leave the last stunted trees behind, reach the outlet of Evolution Lake, and find a few small campsites north of the lake's outlet. The habitat here is ideal for the white-tailed ptarmigan, an introduced species whose population remarkably stabilized at relatively low numbers.

For a short distance, you find yourself walking on sand patches between granite slabs and rocky outcrops. Shortly after the tree cover thickens, you reach the first switchback. This marks the unsigned junction with a use trail to spectacular Darwin Bench, well worth a detour to camp or eat lunch, or, alternatively, to the popular cross-country route up over Lamarck Col. You will now begin a steep descent into Evolution Valley. If you look at the elevation profile between Muir Pass and the Piute Creek junction, you will note that the section can be divided into three "flat" sections, broken by two much steeper descents. First is the section you have just completed: the long, shallow descent through Evolution Basin, a hanging valley. This is now truncated by the descent that lies ahead. Soon you will find yourself in Evolution Valley, another hanging valley. At its end, you will descend steeply to Goddard Canyon. A hanging valley forms when the glacier in the side valley cannot erode its valley floor as quickly as does the glacier in the main valley, creating a steep drop-off. At the first step, the drainage to the McGee Lakes was more eroded than Evolution Basin, and at the second, Goddard Canyon was eroded more quickly than Evolution Valley.

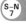

At the base of the grade, you pass a small campsite on open slab and shortly ford the multibranched stream that drains Darwin Canyon— not difficult, but potentially cumbersome. Your route is largely within dry lodgepole forest with occasional excursions to the edge of meadows or onto granite slabs. In the openings, Parish's yampah, alpineflames, and pussytoes are common constituents. Continuing your gradual descent and crossing several tributaries, you reach Colby Meadow and more campsites. Farther along is McClure Meadow, where a summer ranger is stationed. After you pass the first large campsites and two small streams, look north of the trail for the path to the ranger's cabin

[9640' – 5.2/9.9]. The campsites fringing McClure Meadow are justifiably popular for the views they offer—to the west lies a steep monolith, the Hermit, while along the eastern skyline are a handful of the Evolution Basin peaks, Mt. Mendel, Mt. Darwin, Mt. Spencer, and Mt. Huxley. You continue down Evolution Valley, passing occasional campsites and tracing the northern edge of Evolution Meadow. The forest floor is mostly dry, but occasionally, small seeps and tributaries make the ground muddy underfoot. Cassin's finches, with red heads and streaked pinkish backs, and red crossbills, somewhat larger and with the eponymous crossed beaks, are both present in this forest. The JMT presently leads to a creek crossing [9200' – 2.4/12.3]. This crossing fell out of favor some years back when a hole formed around a large rock in the channel. However, except under very high water, it is now safe to cross here again, and the rangers request that you do just that. Otherwise, you will have to backtrack upstream in search of a safer location.

As you continue down valley, the slope increases and, suddenly, you are walking alongside foaming cascades and deep, rounded holes. The grade then becomes dramatically steeper, and you leave the granite behind to enter dark, metamorphic rock, still part of the Goddard Terrane, and descend switchbacks down a steep, west-facing slope into Goddard Canyon. As you descend, stop and enjoy the panoramic vista and especially look across to the west canyon wall. Note the streams and waterfalls flowing down deeply incised and nearly straight fractures in the metamorphic rock; granite rarely forms such straight, narrow channels down a cliff face. At their base, the trail enters a lodgepole forest, passes a large campsite, and then hooks briefly south to a log footbridge crossing the South Fork of the San Joaquin. On its far side, you a reach a junction with the Goddard Canyon/Hell For Sure Pass Trail [8480' – 1.5/ 13.8] and turn north, downcanyon. Just beyond is an easy, but possibly shoes-off creek crossing, and you then traipse alongside a small stream, beside which grow Kelley's tiger lilies, swamp onions, and arrowleaf groundsel, with heads of small, straggly looking, yellow, daisy-like flowers and large leaves shaped like acute triangles. For some distance, you now walk through a relatively moist lodgepole forest before emerging from tree cover at a handsome bridge. Just before you cross, you pass a use trail to some campsites a bit north of the trail.

The steep-walled gorge of fractured metamorphic rocks along which you are now walking is strikingly different from the smooth granite slabs in Evolution Valley and Evolution Basin. You continue downstream, taking in the impressive canyon walls and the turbulent waters of the South Fork of the San Joaquin River. Common species on the dry slope you are traversing include western eupatorium, small-leaved cream bush, granite gilia, and scarlet penstemon. You re-enter forest cover as you approach Aspen Meadow, now a forest that is a mixture of quaking aspen, lodgepole pine, white fir, and the occasional western juniper. There are several campsites within this forested stretch. Before long, you are again in the open, traversing across the dry, sunny, southwest canyon wall. Often far below the trail, the green waters of the river roll and tumble over ledges of dark, metamorphic rock. Both early and late in the day, this is a wonderful place for bird-watching. A Townsend's solitaire may be perched atop one of the western junipers or flying above the stream in search of insects. This brown bird is identified by its melodious song and the yellow-beige pattern visible on its wings when it flies. Swarms of violet-green swallows also dive playfully above the water. By midseason, rufous hummingbirds are likely sucking nectar from the abundant flowers. At night, bats emerge, likely from crevices in the steep metamorphic wall to the west, to feed on insects. Before long, you pass numerous well-used campsites on a large, Jeffrey pine-shaded flat, and cross turbulent Piute Creek on a steel footbridge, leaving behind Kings Canyon National Park and entering John Muir Wilderness. On the far side of the footbridge, you reach a junction with the Piute Pass Trail, which goes north through Humphreys Basin and over Piute Pass to North Lake [8050′ – 3.5/17.3].

The JMT diverges from the river, crossing over open, rocky, dry knobs of metamorphic rock with sedge meadows and scattered western junipers and Jeffrey pines. Take your time to enjoy the majestic trees. This open, flat valley of dark-colored rock is markedly different from anything you have seen to the south, or anything you will see to the north. Northern flicker's can be common at these elevations. This species of woodpecker feeds mostly on the ground and is easily identified by its red-orange underwings, visible in flight.

Near where forest cover resumes, you reach a junction with the Florence Lake Trail, here referred to as the "southern JMT cutoff" [7880′ – 1.8/19.1]. It is thus known because this is the cutoff northbound JMT hikers take to reach either the Muir Trail Ranch, a food-drop depot, or Florence Lake (see Appendix B for further route description). The hot pool at Blayney Hot Springs is also accessed by this trail, but crossing the San Joaquin to reach the hot springs can be dangerous, or impossible, during high flow. Passing the halfway point between Whitney Portal and Yosemite Valley, the JMT now begins a traversing ascent, mostly through open Jeffrey pine forest, to reach a second junction that leads to the Florence Lake Trail near the Muir Trail Ranch, the "northern JMT cutoff" [8400' – 1.7/20.8]. If you have left the trail to pick up a food cache and do not too much mind missing a short stretch of the JMT, this is the junction where you will continue your northward journey on the JMT.

You now begin a long, dry climb up a scrubby, south-facing slope. The grade is continuous, with no benches for camping. Near the bottom, you are mostly under tree cover of Jeffrey pines with scattered western junipers. Higher up, you emerge onto an open slope, covered with greenleaf manzanita and mountain whitethorn, a shrub with intimidating thorns and small, blue-green leaves. A collection of herbs, including wavy-leaved paintbrush, pennyroyal, and Anderson's thistle exist as an understory. Fox sparrows enjoy this vegetation and may be seen hopping in and out of the bushes. The switchbacks enter open lodgepole forest a short distance before you reach Senger Creek [9740' – 2.1/22.9]. Note that some areas on either side of the crossing may have "no camping" signs, either for restoration or because they are too close to water, but legal campsites exist as well.

Another bout of switchbacks, including a section passing large, chinquapin-covered boulders, brings you to a very marshy meadow and a small creek, a fork of Senger Creek. A short distance onward, beneath lodgepole pine cover, are a couple of nice campsites. Farther up, the JMT curves southeast through a meadow before crossing the outlet to the Sallie Keyes Lakes on a logjam. To the right of the trail, near the meadow, is a snow survey cabin, at which a ranger is sometimes stationed. There are many large campsites beneath lodgepole cover as you follow the west shore of the lower Sallie Keyes Lake. A row of especially impressive lodgepole pines lines the bank of the lake; they are uncrowded and artistic, as if each were intentionally placed. The trail crosses Sallie Keyes Creek between the two lakes and climbs beyond the upper lake. The trail now switchbacks upward, crosses the outlet stream several more times, reaches Heart Lake, and skirts along its eastern shore. Small parties can camp at an exposed site with open views near Heart Lake's outlet. From here, the trail ascends both sandy, dry slopes, and wetter ones, along seeps or small patches of meadow. One common species on the sandy slopes is spreading phlox, with a woody base, crawling stems, and needle-like leaves. Its white, five-petal flowers are tubular at their base, with petal tips that extend outward at right angles. These switchbacks pass quickly, and before long, you will be taking a breather atop the pass, an almost quaint gap between granite walls and boulders [10,890' – 3.6/26.5].

SEE MAP 7

SECTION 6.

Selden Pass to Silver Pass—Mono and Bear Creeks

Once you cross the divide, you can look northward at the Mono Recesses. As you descend, be sure to stop and enjoy the vista, which improves a few switchbacks below Selden Pass, with exquisite views of Marie Lake, framed by the peaks crowning the Mono Recesses. The impressive pyramidal peak to the east is Seven Gables, whose shape is even more awe-inspiring when viewed from the north. This pass is much lower than those to the south, and the first trees appear quickly. Before long, you reach Marie Lake, which fills a large, shallow basin trimmed with and underlain by granite slabs, creating an oddly shaped lake dotted with islands. Several open campsites, some with vistas northward, can be found on sandy patches near the outlet [10,540′ – 0.9/0.9].

The trail now descends again, entering a zone with scattered whitebark pines and mountain hemlocks. These short-needled conifers with small, elongate cones are much more common in the northern Sierra,

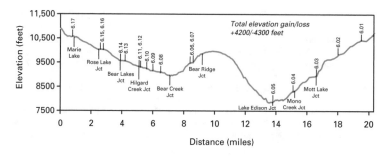

and even there, they prefer cooler, north-facing slopes. This is, in fact, the first time the JMT passes through a stand of them; to the south, they were only present in steep, north-facing draws. But I leave it to John Muir to further describe his favorite tree: "The hemlock spruce is the most singularly beautiful of all the California coniferæ. So slender is its axis at the top that it bends over and droops like the stalk of a nodding lily. The branches droop also, and divide into innumerable slender, waving sprays, which are arranged in a varied, eloquent harmony that is wholly indescribable." Be sure to spend one night on your walk beneath their elegant boughs. En route, you also pass a few large glacial erratics, notable because dark-colored rock fragments are embedded in an otherwise light-colored granite. This is rock from a small outcrop to the southwest that was transported downslope by a glacier.

The next campsites you reach are some distance later, on slabs just above Rosemarie Meadow. Here is also the junction with a trail that climbs southwest to Rose Lake [10,035' – 1.6/2.5], where you will find good, secluded camping. Lemmon's paintbrush, dwarf bilberry, primrose monkeyflower, and bog kalmia are all common species here. Bog kalmia has flowers similar to red heather, but it forms upright carpets

Location	Elevation	Distance from Previous Point	Cumulative Distance	UTM Coordinates
Selden Pass	10,890	—	0	11S 334070E 4128460N
Marie Lake outlet	10,540	0.9	0.9	11S 334218E 4129774N
Rose Lake junction	10,035	1.6	2.5	11S 334195E 4131442N
Three Island Lake junction	10,015	0.3	2.8	11S 334429E 4131706N
Bear Lakes junction	9570	1.1	3.9	11S 334661E 4132955N
Hilgard Fork junction	9320	1.2	5.1	11S 333898E 4134673N
Bear Creek junction	8970	2.0	7.1	11S 332858E 4137219N
Bear Ridge junction	9880	2.1	9.2	11S 330945E 4138822N
Lake Edison junction	7900	4.6	13.8	11S 329758E 4142189N
Mono Creek junction	8350	1.4	15.2	11S 331029E 4143228N
Mott Lake junction	8980	1.4	16.6	11S 331341E 4145024N
Silver Pass	10,750	3.7	20.3	11S 330017E 4148322N

SEE MAP 7

in flat, marshy areas and has larger leaves. If you turn around here, you will have excellent views of pyramid-shaped Mt. Hooper, west of Selden Pass. Just a tad farther north, you meet a trail that departs east for Three Island Lake and Lou Beverly Lake [10,015' – 0.3/2.8], where there are additional campsites. Within 200 yards of this junction, you first pass one small campsite and then cross the West Fork of Bear Creek on a large log.

The trail now descends through dry lodgepole forest toward a notoriously deep and potentially dangerous ford across Bear Creek. This crossing is made particularly difficult early season, since the swift water is often combined with swarms of mosquitoes in the area. However, by late season, flow has decreased and the abundant western blueberry bushes lining the banks of the stream may yield an appetizing snack. Beyond the crossing is a junction with the trail that leads up the East Fork of Bear Creek [9570' – 1.1/3.9]. Continuing downstream, you pass through a marshier area (if you are having difficulty following the trail, it trends to the right), and then through denser lodgepole forest. You soon cross multistranded Hilgard Creek, likely a wade for the first crossing during high flow and over logs on the other two. There are campsites to either side of the trio of crossings. Just beyond the crossing, you reach the Hilgard Fork Trail junction, leading up to Lake Italy and then over Italy Pass on an unmaintained trail [9320' – 1.2/5.1].

Soon begins a beautiful section of Bear Creek, in stretches lined by granite slabs and containing enticing swimming holes when the water is low. The JMT descends through lodgepole-dominated forest, passing numerous campsites. In places, the forest gives way to openings of dry sedge meadows. In these, Parish's yampah, pretty faces, and Leichtlin's mariposa lily are all common. Pretty faces, often growing in dense masses, are pale yellow, six-petal flowers related to lilies. Leichtlin's mariposa lily are three-petal, mostly white flowers that generally grow individually; *mariposa* is the Spanish word for butterfly, and the petals of many mariposa lilies indeed look like brightly colored wings. Before long, you reach the Bear Creek Trail junction [8970' – 2.0/7.1]. This track leads to the Lake Thomas Edison area via the Bear Diversion Dam, providing the shortest access to the post office at Mono Hot Springs and, less directly, the Vermilion Valley Resort (see Appendix B).

You now leave the shores of rollicking Bear Creek and begin a climb up to Bear Ridge. Gaining little elevation at first, the trail continues north across a wet slope, with many small stream crossings and muddy sections. Slowly, you begin climbing up a slope dotted by beautiful western junipers. About halfway up the slope, alongside an unmapped stream and beneath Jeffrey pines, is a beautiful campsite. Other possibilities exist a bit farther along, on small, exposed, sandy flats. These are your last campsites until you reach Mono Creek on the far side of Bear Ridge. As you climb, be sure to turn around for a beautiful vista north to Seven Gables. To the west of the main summit is its sub-peak, with the seven namesake gables or ridges, running longitudinally down its north face. On one of the final switchbacks, you pass a small seep covered by wildflowers and dense vegetation–enjoy it and fill your water bottles, as the next many miles are quite dry. Just beyond, you reach the junction with the Bear Ridge Trail, another alternative to reach Lake Thomas Edison [9880' – 2.1/9.2], and also the starting point for a detour to Volcanic Knob (see Appendix E).

This long, flat section of trail heads north across Bear Ridge, through pure lodgepole pine stands. As you descend toward Mono Creek, you will pass through many different types of forest stands, with species composition that is a function of elevation, moisture, and soil texture. Ground cover is variable throughout the climb, but nearly always sparse, with rock cress, alpine prickly currant, and creeping snowberry, the most common species. Creeping snowberry is a sprawling vine identified by its small, pink, tubular flowers and slightly lobed leaves. As the grade increases, the forest becomes a mix of lodgepole and western white pines. Western white pine has mid-sized needles in groups of five, arranged on the branch to give them an airy appearance. Decreasing elevations gives way to a forest of western white pines, red firs, and mountain hemlocks. A bit lower, white firs dominate the forest. And finally, at the base of the climb, western white pines, lodgepole pines, and a few western junipers grow together. Compared to red fir, white fir has much longer needles and often paler bark. Its cones differ as well, but these are always consumed by critters before dropping from the trees, and therefore are of little use to hikers for identification. Finally, many, many switchbacks later, the trail crosses first a small tributary, and then Mono Creek, on a steel footbridge just beyond the junction with the Lake Edison Trail [7900' – 4.6/13.8]. This trail leads you to Quail Meadows and the Lake Edison ferry landing and the Vermilion Valley Resort, a hospitable resupply stop for JMT and PCT travelers (see Appendix B). There is camping both near the trail junction beneath majestic Jeffrey pines, and a short distance off the JMT in Quail Meadows.

The climbing resumes yet again, now toward Silver Pass. The forest consists of towering Jeffrey pines, occasional western junipers, and stands of white fir. Shortly, you ford the North Fork of Mono Creek for

SEE MAP 8

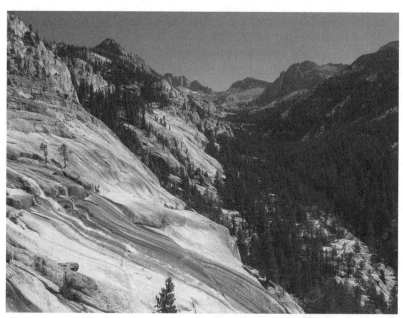

A cascading waterfall to the north of the Mott Lake Trail junction

the first of many times. The water flow may be high and difficult, but at least the river bottom is flat, broad, and covered with small pebbles. As you follow the river course upstream, note a few campsites in openings beneath stands of Jeffrey pines. At the junction with the Mono Pass Trail [8350' – 1.4/15.2], the JMT turns north and the grade becomes steeper. Cross through stretches of mixed conifer forest and traverse open slabs dotted with western junipers, and then begin a climb up dry, rocky switchbacks. Stretches dominated by quaking aspens are indicative of regular disturbance, usually from avalanches. They are the first tree species to re-grow following such disturbance and often continue to grow even after being flattened by recurring avalanches. The bright blue, tubular flowers of showy penstemon greet you throughout the ascent. Where the grade next eases, you enter lush Pocket Meadow, filled with the tall, yellow, sunflower-like flowers of orange sneezeweed. Just beyond, you reach a small campsite and the junction with the trail to Mott Lake [8980' – 1.4/16.6]

The next crossing, another ford of the North Fork of Mono Creek, is one of the most dangerous along the JMT, as the creekbed is filled with boulders and the water is turbulent, making footing difficult. This crossing should not be done in bare feet. You proceed up many switchbacks to the hanging valley above. The vegetation here, which always

SEE MAP 8

dominates dry, sandy, south-facing slopes, is now very familiar to you. Partway up the slope, the trail fords Silver Pass Creek. This can be a dangerous crossing because of the dashing cascades above and below you. With luck, though, a series of well-placed boulders will be above the water that you can use to carefully work your way across. Having to make two such wretched crossings, one right after the other, seems very unfair. As you round the corner atop the last switchback, turn around and look down into the valley out of which you just climbed. Take a brief break to enjoy the waterfall and beautiful granite slabs to your right (east). A bit farther along, the track skirts the southwestern edge of a large meadow with a meandering stream whose edges are lined by western bistort, with tall stalks and dense heads of small, white flowers. This species becomes an ever more dominant member of meadow communities as you continue north. Before long, you have another (easier) ford across Silver Pass Creek and pass several campsites under open lodgepole cover. Alongside outcropping rock, the clusters of dense-flowered spiraea are likely to catch your attention. You ascend benches with decreasing forest cover, interspersed with openings surrounding granite slabs.

The trail climbs to Silver Pass Lake, although the lake lies sufficiently west of the trail that it isn't initially visible. Nonetheless, if you head west where the trail flattens, you will find several sandy tent sites nestled among the lodgepole pines at the southeast end of the lake. Ahead are long stretches of open, sandy flats, inhabited by Belding's ground squirrels, a species resembling miniature groundhogs in shape and in behavior, as they stand upright and stare at you from their burrow entrances. Higher again, you cross small, alpine meadows, dotted with mountain paintbrush, a meadow-dwelling paintbrush with red and yellow flowers. They are covered in small glands that sparkle in the sun. If you look westward as you climb the last slope to the pass, you will enjoy a peek at a small pothole lake with sapphire blue water. The true pass (and drainage divide) across the Silver Divide [10,750′ – 3.7/20.3] is two switchbacks below the trail's high point. The JMT climbs up a higher shoulder to bypass a cliff on the north side of Silver Pass.

SEE MAP 8

SECTION 5.

Silver Pass to Fresno-Madera County Line—Fish Creek Fork of the Middle Fork of the San Joaquin River

Descending north from the shoulder above Silver Pass is the last time you will be able to enjoy alpine scenery until you approach Donohue Pass, many miles to the north. In the far distance are two dark, steep peaks, Mt. Ritter and Banner Peak, whose bases you will pass in a few days. Through much of the season, there may be a small, though quite steep, snow bank down the first 50 feet of the shoulder, but it is easily navigated or bypassed. You descend toward Chief Lake on shallow, sandy slopes dotted with stunted whitebark pines. When water is present, there are many exposed campsites between Silver Pass and Chief Lake, all with excellent views. Frosted buckwheat, alpine paintbrush, spreading phlox, and Nuttall's sandwort are all common here.

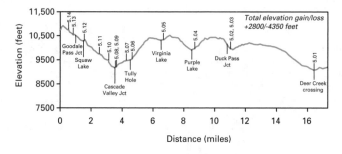

Passing the junction to the Goodale Pass Trail [10,530' − 1.0/1.0], you descend more steeply toward exquisitely placed Squaw Lake, whose outlet you cross on large solid rocks. This small lake, surrounded by alpine meadows and steep cliffs, has several small campsites just northeast of its outlet [10,300' − 0.5/1.5].

Descending, you enter more continuous forest cover, ever more dominated by mountain hemlocks. Around 9700 feet, you pass around the shores of a beautiful little marshy meadow, alongside which there is one campsite amongst open trees. You cross its outlet stream on a small footbridge, and shortly thereafter, you cross it again in a lupine-covered opening, before entering a magical forest of dense mountain hemlocks and lodgepole pines. The thick tree cover undoubtedly feels odd in the Sierra, where you nearly always have a filtered view through the trees. Occasional benches to the west of the trail provide small campsites, ringed by heath vegetation: dwarf bilberries, red mountain heather, western Labrador tea, and white mountain heather. Labrador tea, which, despite its name, is poisonous, is a shrub with white flowers and leathery leaves. White mountain heather, one of John Muir's favorites, has flowers that are shaped like little white bells with red caps. As for birdlife, black-eyed juncos and American robins are likely present around the tree bases.

Location	Elevation	Distance from Previous Point	Cumulative Distance	UTM Coordinates
Silver Pass	10,750	—	0	11S 330017E 4148322N
Goodale Pass junction	10,530	1.0	1.0	11S 329472E 4149131N
Squaw Lake outlet	10,300	0.5	1.5	11S 329950E 4149412N
Cascade Creek junction	9190	2.0	3.5	11S 329182E 4150922N
Tully Hole junction	9520	1.0	4.5	11S 329943E 4152061N
Lake Virginia inlet	10,338	2.0	6.5	11S 329261E 4153679N
Purple Lake outlet	9925	2.0	8.5	11S 327825E 4154989N
Duck Pass junction	10,170	2.3	10.8	11S 326105E 4156217N
Deer Creek crossing	9100	5.6	16.4	11S 320455E 4159144N
Madera-Fresno County Line	9220	0.9	17.3	11S 319953E 4160145N

SEE MAP 8

Shortly, you reach the junction with the trail down Cascade Valley [9190' – 2.0/ 3.5]. This trail junction, nestled amid avalanche debris, is not always obviously marked, so make sure you take the right fork that begins the climb toward Tully Hole. This junction may be particularly confusing: Many maps, including the USGS 7.5-minute topos, show that the trail crosses the drainage you have been following before the trail junction, and that the trail junction is therefore farther downstream. In fact, the trail you have been following always remains to the east of the side drainage.

Just northwest the junction, you pass one campsite on a knob and another a short distance later, beyond a small creek crossing. You now emerge from the forest, cross Fish Creek on a steel footbridge, and climb up a steep slope with picturesque western junipers and abundant Leichtlin's mariposa lilies. Where the slope lessens, you enter a lodgepole forest and follow it alongside Fish Creek, enjoying beautiful sections of slab and deep swimming holes. En route, you pass a few campsites before reaching Tully Hole and a junction with the trail that crosses Fish Creek to climb eastward up to McGee Pass [9520' – 1.0/4.5]. Just beyond this junction is a large campsite used by pack groups. Now you begin a climb up an open slope toward Lake Virginia. Near the beginning of this climb, you approach a few little streams. Note the abundant vegetation: great red paintbrush, Coulter's daisy, Sierra rein orchid, and much more. You climb switchbacks up the increasingly dry, sandy slope and begin to pass shaggy hawkweed, scarlet penstemon, Anderson's thistles, pennyroyal, and the wavy-leaved paintbrush.

At the top of the switchbacks, the trail curves westward, passes over a broad, sandy saddle, and descends gradually to Lake Virginia. Just before the lake, you pass a small stand of lodgepole pines. This is a good place to see mountain chickadees, as the trees here have low branches where you may see the little birds, which hang upside down as they feed. You can always tell when these birds are nearby by their *chick-a-dee-dee* call; one higher, shorter note, followed by two lower, longer ones. The meadows surrounding Lake Virginia's inlet provide wonderful places to take a break [10,338' – 2.0/6.5]. Lemmon's paintbrush, mountain paintbrush, and little elephant's heads are all abundant and create a colorful meadow surrounding the lovely, large, subalpine lake, which has open views to the south. There are campsites amongst scattered trees on the sandy knob to the northwest of the lake.

From Lake Virginia, climb to another sandy saddle, atop which is another rock glacier and one of the last steep, craggy faces that were so common farther south. Large patches of long-stemmed, five-petal, white

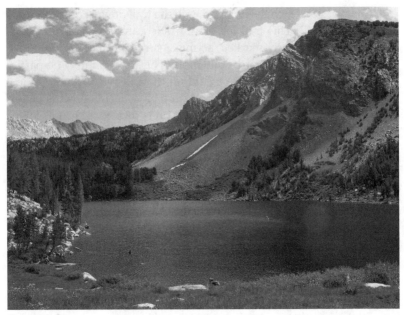

Purple Lake

flowers with mousetail-like stalks of leaves may stand out. These are mousetail ivesia. Spreading phlox, granite gilia, and Sierra penstemon are also common. As you then descend switchbacks into dry lodgepole forests, you first pass carpets of Sierra arnica and then increasingly find yourself staring at bare forest floor. The grade next eases are you approach beautiful Purple Lake. In the past, the ford across Purple Lake's outlet stream could be difficult, but a new bridge makes for an easy crossing. Camping is prohibited within 300 feet of the outlet. Just beyond the outlet, the JMT passes a junction that leads down into Cascade Valley [9925' – 2.0/8.5], and a short distance later, it passes a use trail that leads north to campsites on the west shore of Purple Lake.

Leaving Purple Lake behind, the trail climbs just a short distance and begins an open traverse westward. There are few trees along this south-facing slope, and you have a beautiful view of the walls of glaciated Cascade Valley. If you turn around, you can look southeast toward Mt. Abbot, a peak on the Sierra Crest. Although it is dry, many flowers dot the granite soil, the same collection of species that is common on most dry slopes. After some distance, you pass over a small saddle and descend slightly into Duck Creek's valley, shortly reaching the junction with the trail over Duck Pass [10,170' – 2.3/10.8]. Your decent continues to Duck Creek, a ford that is not dangerous, but under high water, it is likely a wade. Beyond the creek, there are a few campsites clustered amongst granite slabs, some of which are visible from the trail. Others can be found by following the western bank downstream. Be sure to fill your water bottles at Duck Creek, as the next reliable water is at Deer Creek, more than 5 miles away.

To many, the next section is among the most monotonous on the JMT: Until you approach Deer Creek, the vegetation and views change little. But pay close attention to a change in rock type, as this traverse begins on granite cobble and gravel and ends in soft, but dusty pumice sand, through which you will be walking for the next many miles. Openings in the forest provide occasional glimpses south to the Silver Divide. And as you meander through the lodgepole forest, you are likely to see several bird species. In addition to the ubiquitous dark-eyed juncos, these forests are home to the blue grouse, often perched high in the trees. In early summer, the *whoop-whoop-whoop* of the males, followed by a sudden flurry of wing beats, is likely to startle you. You may also see red-breasted nuthatches that have straight, chisel-like bills, and the curved-billed brown creeper. The former circle down, and the latter circle up tree trunks in search of insects. For long distances, the forest floor is nearly bare, with only rock cress and western wallflower growing. Openings in the forest sport a few shrubs, including mountain sagebrush and bush chinquapin. While only lodgepole pines can survive under the dry conditions dictated by the southern exposure, especially in conjunction with coarse, volcanic soils, as you approach Deer Creek, western white pines appear as well. Finally, you reach the Deer Creek ford [9100' – 5.6/16.4], to either side of which are a number of campsites frequented by stock parties. Just beyond, the JMT passes an indistinct and unmarked junction with a lateral up Deer Creek, and the JMT climbs gently through open lodgepole forest to a sandy saddle and unlikely drainage divide. This point, the Fresno-Madera County line, marks the boundary between the main Middle Fork of the San Joaquin drainage and Fish Creek [9220' – 0.9/17.3].

SEE MAP 9

SECTION 4.

Fresno-Madera County Line to Island Pass—Middle Fork of the San Joaquin River

The JMT now crunches north-northwest over pumice, crossing a small fork of Crater Creek, and then Crater Creek itself, en route to Upper Crater Meadow. Several tracks leave the meadow, all headed toward Mammoth Pass. The first (southernmost) of these tracks is the main one [8915' – 1.1/1.1]. Campsites can be found in the forested fringes around the meadow. Your gentle descent continues north down a small ravine, crossing Crater Creek again, reaching Crater Meadow, and crossing Crater Creek one final time, on a fallen log, in the vicinity of the two Red Cones. There are several campsites on the south side of Crater Creek and one a short distance up the northern Red Cone. Along the stream banks, a short distance below the crossing, a few, mostly collapsed, lava tubes are visible. On the north side of the crossing is a

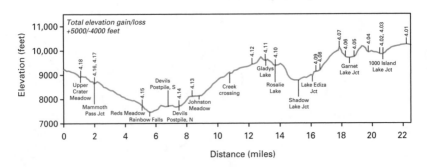

SEE MAP 9

little-used and poorly marked junction with a trail northeast to Mammoth Pass [8645′ – 0.9/2.0].

An ascent of one or both of the Red Cones is highly recommended (see Appendix E). The vista from the summit not only lets you gaze over the country you will cover between now and Donohue Pass, but you also get a close-up view of Mammoth Mountain. A bit of geologic history: The volcanic activity of the last 3 million years formed the pumice deposits you have walked over and will continue to walk over.

Location	Elevation	Distance from Previous Point	Cumulative Distance	UTM Coordinates
Madera-Fresno County Line	9220	—	0	11S 319953E 4160145N
Mammoth Pass junction in Upper Crater Meadow	8915	1.1	1.1	11S 319252E 4161498N
Crater Creek crossing at Red Cones	8645	0.9	2.0	11S 318338E 4162253N
Reds Meadow junction	7715	3.1	5.1	11S 316900E 4164357N
Rainbow Falls junction	7475	0.5	5.6	11S 316244E 4164846N
Southern Devils Postpile junction	7710	1.2	6.8	11S 315855E 4165917N
Northern Devils Postpile junction	7685	0.7	7.5	11S 315747E 4166939N
Beck Lakes junction	8090	0.7	8.2	11S 315353E 4167777N
Johnston Meadow	8120	0.6	8.8	11S 314827E 4168538N
Trinity Lakes outlet crossing	9045	2.0	10.8	11S 314721E 4170195N
Gladys Lake	9575	2.3	13.1	11S 313189E 4172430N
Rosalie Lake outlet	9350	0.6	13.7	11S 313028E 4173139N
Shadow Lake junction	8760	1.5	15.2	11S 311695E 4173764N
Lake Ediza junction	9000	0.9	16.1	11S 311088E 4173423N
Garnet Lake junction	9680	2.4	18.5	11S 310475E 4176159N
Thousand Island Lake junction	9830	2.2	20.7	11S 308736E 4177715N
Island Pass	10,205	1.8	22.5	11S 306699E 4178705N

About 760,000 years ago, an enormous eruption formed Long Valley Caldera, a bit east of the Sierra, depositing ash as far east as Nebraska. At 220,000 years, Mammoth Mountain, a dormant volcano, is a more recent addition. These events are separate from the much older volcanic events that led to the formation of the Ritter Range. Those dark rocks to the west likely resulted from a catastrophic caldera collapse 100 million years ago, and were metamorphosed during the events that led to the emplacement of the underlying granite. Today, Mammoth Mountain is, of course, best known as an enormous ski area that receives enormous quantities of snow. This is no coincidence, as the passes crossing the Sierra Crest in this vicinity are the lowest for a great distance north and south, allowing storms that are elsewhere blocked by tall mountains to funnel straight to the slopes of Mammoth Mountain. The ski area founder had done his homework: He was previously a snow surveyor.

The JMT now makes a switchbacking descent toward Devils Postpile, along the Middle Fork of the San Joaquin River. You complete much of the descent under forest cover—a combination of Jeffrey pines, western junipers, western white pines, and white firs—before suddenly emerging on a burnt slope, the result of the Rainbow Fire, a large, lightning-caused forest fire in 1992. As you descend this shrubby slope, you cross four branches of Boundary Creek; the banks of each are colored by dense vegetation. Although the dusty pumice substrate might be even less appealing without forest cover, the open slopes display abundant bird life, including yellow-rumped warblers, mountain bluebirds, and swallows, as well as a community of plants that only thrive following burns. As you gaze at the thick, spiny shrubs on either side of the trail, you will be thankful to be on a maintained trail. Two of the more vicious shrubs are Sierra gooseberries, with 1-centimeter-wide, spiny (but otherwise tasty) berries, and mountain whitethorn. Due to the steep slope and abundant undergrowth, there are no camping options between the Red Cones and Reds Meadow Resort.

Turning right at the first junction [7715' – 3.1/5.1], you most efficiently reach Reds Meadow Resort, where you may have a food parcel to retrieve, or wish to eat at the cafe, fill your water bottles, or buy additional supplies (see Appendix B for details). There are also campgrounds near the Reds Meadow Resort, as well as at Devils Postpile National Monument, about a mile to the north (however, only at Reds Meadow are there showers and sites specially reserved for backpackers). Both locations also provide access to the shuttlebus, which runs every 30 minutes midseason and travels to the Mammoth Mountain ski area, your gateway to the town of Mammoth Lakes. Over the next

SEE MAPS 9–10

half mile, you will pass three more junctions, the first two providing alternative routes north to Reds Meadow Resort, and the third heading toward Devils Postpile National Monument [7475' – 0.5/5.6]. From this third junction, you can also detour south to Rainbow Falls if you have the time and energy.

Side Trip: Devils Postpile

If you have not previously visited Devils Postpile, I recommend a detour to this geologic attraction, since the JMT provides only fleeting and distant glances of the formation.

At the third junction, leave the JMT and head north for approximately 1 mile, staying left where you pass another junction. Shortly, you reach yet another junction, the southern tip of a loop around Devils Postpile.

Now a bit of geologic background: Devils Postpile formed less than 100,000 years ago, following an eruption of basaltic magma. Slow, even cooling conditions, and magma with a consistent chemical composition throughout allowed the hexagonal columns to form. Because of the topography, an unusually deep flow of magma accumulated, such that the interior was well insulated and cooled slowly and evenly. As magma cools, it contracts and hence must fracture. Physics dictates that fractures 120 degrees apart most efficiently release building stress, leading to hexagonal columns. Devils Postpile is one of the tallest and most nearly perfect examples of columnar basalt in the world.

Be sure to walk around the loop, as it takes you both to the top of the formation, where glacially polished tops of columns are exposed, and to the base of the formation, where you can gaze up at the columns and gawk at the talus field of hexagonal-shaped rocks. At the end of your detour, continue north from the northern end of the loop. Take the next junction you encounter, with a trail that trends southwest to the riverbank. Cross the Middle Fork of the San Joaquin River on a footbridge and head north to intersect the JMT.

Those skipping Devils Postpile should continue west along the JMT, shortly crossing the Middle Fork of the San Joaquin on a footbridge. Now trending north, you continue through the area denuded by the Rainbow Fire. If you find yourself annoyed by the pumice's dusty nature, stop and appreciate how soft it is underfoot. As before, the wildflower displays can be astonishing, and the aerial antics of the abundant swallows engaging. Shortly, you begin a gentle climb up a dusty track across a steep pumice slope. You pass an X-junction, where a spur from Devils Postpile crosses the JMT and heads southwest toward King Creek [7710' – 1.2/6.8]. The JMT continues to the northwest. You are now walking past the postpiles, but with the exception of one knob, they are hidden from view. You then reach a second X-junction, where those who detoured to Devils Postpile will rejoin the JMT [7685' – 0.7/7.5]. At this point, the PCT and JMT, which have followed the same path since just beyond Crabtree Meadow, diverge; the PCT takes a more easterly route for the next 12 miles.

Now exiting Devils Postpile National Monument, you continue up a dry, open, pumice slope. You next reach a junction with a trail west to Beck Lakes [8090' – 0.7/8.2], and just beyond cross Minaret Creek on a log bridge. This enticing pebble-bottomed creek would be a wonderful place to cool your feet. Beneath scattered tree cover, the JMT passes a few campsites and continues across loose pumice soils to a T-junction with a trail that goes northwest to Minaret Lake [8120' – 0.6/8.8]. Southwest of the junction, the JMT trends right to begin a steeper climb northward. Across the trail are boggy Johnston Meadow and little Johnston Lake. Most of your ascent is on a dry, sandy, pumice slope, with Anderson's thistles and pennyroyal among the most common species, but occasionally you cross a small seep and encounter a wetter plant community. Red fir, western white pines, and a few lodgepole pines grow overhead; shortly, the red fir will disappear and only re-appear on the final descent into Yosemite Valley. As this forest is lower in elevation than many along the JMT, it is filled with birdlife: Keep your ears open for a black-backed woodpecker whacking on a dead tree or a northern goshawk screeching as it flies through the forest.

Shortly, the JMT crosses the Trinity Lakes outlet, with a colorful display of wildflowers, including crimson columbine and corn lilies [9045' – 2.0/10.8]. Continuing up Volcanic Ridge, the JMT skirts the marshy Trinity Lakes, now under mountain hemlocks, western white pines, and a few lodgepole pines. If you are willing to walk a few hundred feet to water, there are many sandy campsites on the west side of the trail, but also keep your eyes peeled for campsites closer to water.

SEE MAP 10

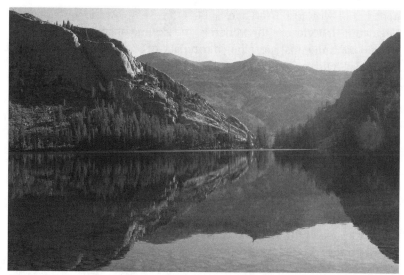

Shadow Lake with the San Joaquin Ridge in the background

The JMT rolls over a little saddle and shortly reaches hemlock-fringed Gladys Lake [9575' – 2.3/13.1], which has a number of good campsites. The trail climbs a little and then dips down to skirt Rosalie Lake's north and east shores, along which there are also some good campsites. There are mountain hemlocks overhead and western Labrador tea underfoot as you approach a logjam across the outlet [9350' – 0.6/13.7]. Leaving shady Rosalie Lake behind, you briefly emerge from the forest, reach a small saddle, and begin a 650-foot descent through dense hemlock forest to picturesque Shadow Lake. At the Shadow Lake inlet, you cross a handsome footbridge and reach another junction: A right turn takes you back down to the Middle Fork of the San Joaquin River and out to Agnew Meadows, while the JMT turns left (west) [8760' – 1.5/15.2]. Along the JMT, camping is prohibited between Shadow Lake and the junction 0.9 mile to the west. If this regulation is relaxed in the future, please still consider camping outside of this very high-use corridor: This is a favorite destination for weekend hikers.

You now begin your next climb, alternately through lodgepole forest and across open, slabby knobs composed of the meta-volcanic rock of the Ritter Range. The fast-flowing stream is a good location to spot an American dipper (also known as a water ouzel), a round, grayish bird that can often be seen diving in and out of rapids in search of insects; its constantly bending knees confirm its identity. Soon you reach a T-junction, where the JMT turns right, while the trail straight ahead takes you to Ediza Lake [9000' – 0.9/16.1]. At the junction, you have your first view of the Minarets, the skyline of spires to the south. As you continue upslope, along a tributary of Shadow Creek, you pass shady flats with good campsites. Before long, the trail becomes steeper, and you ascend a dry slope with an understory of manzanita topped by majestic western junipers—and boasting a fantastic view of the Minarets. Re-entering forest cover, you climb up a tiny canyon, pass a small meadow, and reach a saddle atop a ridge. Here there are a few mediocre tent sites and a swimming-pool-sized pond that warms up enough by midsummer for pleasant bathing. You descend mostly open zigzags toward beautiful, windy Garnet Lake, passing scattered mountain hemlocks, beneath which you may see large tufts of pink heuchera. As you approach the lake, you pass one campsite perched on a small flat to the side of the lake, but note that camping is prohibited within a quarter mile of Garnet Lake's outlet. The JMT then traces Garnet Lake's south shore before reaching a junction with a rough trail that descends northeast into the canyon of the Middle Fork of the San Joaquin River [9680' – 2.4/18.5]. Mt. Ritter and Banner Peak, the high points of the Ritter Range, dominate the view westward. You then cross Garnet Lake's outlet on a footbridge, follow its north shore, passing large patches of red heather, and shortly begin your next climb. Near where the switchbacks begin is one legal campsite; there are others down a use trail along Garnet's northwest shore—the sites get better the farther you go toward Garnet's head.

The JMT now climbs rocky switchbacks to the ridgetop above Ruby Lake. Pretty faces, Sierra penstemon, and wavy-leaved paintbrush are all abundant here. From the saddle, the JMT descends to Ruby Lake, surrounded on the west by impressive walls and to the northeast by enormous mats of manzanita. There are small campsites near the outlet, beneath mountain hemlock cover. Descending again, you pass pretty Emerald Lake, whose western shore is closed to camping, and approach island-dotted Thousand Island Lake, finding campsites on the bluff to the southwest of the lake. As per Garnet Lake, camping is prohibited within a quarter mile of its outlet. While Mt. Ritter and Banner Peak were both visible from Garnet Lake, Banner Peak is now the centerpiece. The view of Banner Peak over Thousand Island Lake is irresistibly photogenic and has been memorialized in many of Ansel Adams' most famous photographs—how appropriate that this area is now part of his namesake wilderness. Continuing to the northeast, you cross Thousand Island Lake's outlet on a footbridge and quickly reach a junction [9830' – 2.2/20.7]. Here, the JMT and PCT merge and will

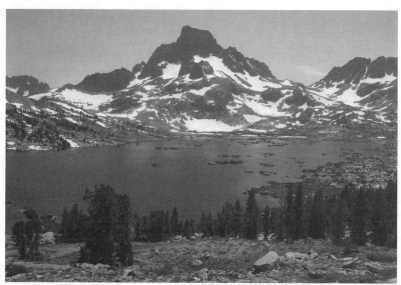

Thousand Island Lake with Banner Peak in the background

again follow the same trail north to Tuolumne Meadows. Meanwhile, heading west from this junction is a use trail around the lake's northwest shore, along which there are many camping options.

You now climb up a dry slope of volcanic soils and slabs. Bright blue mountain bluebirds are common on these bare slopes, perched on snags between insect-catching forays. Western blue flax, which you last saw while descending from Mt. Whitney, is present here, and there are large masses of pretty faces. As you approach the summit of Island Pass, take one last look southward at the dark Ritter Range; before long, you will be back in granite, and the mountains will change in character. Shortly, the climb ends amid dry meadows and many marshy tarns atop Island Pass. The unmarked high point is toward the northern end of the plateau [10,205' – 1.8/22.5]. There are many small campsites amongst the ponds.

SECTION 3.

Island Pass to Donohue Pass—Rush Creek

The next 4.9-mile stretch to the top of Donohue Pass is the only leg of the JMT that is east of the Sierra Crest. Rush Creek drains into Mono Lake, the famous Great Basin salt lake with no outlet. As you begin your descent, you cross over a small seep, but then begin switchbacking down through dry, lodgepole forest. Pussytoes, pussypaws, and Sierra penstemon are three of the only plants to grace the coarse, meta-volcanic soils. Before long, you reach an area known as the Rush Creek Forks, named from the many creek crossings, the more difficult of which all have log bridges. You first pass the Davis Lakes Trail junction [9680' – 1.0/1.0], and next reach the Rush Creek Trail junction [9640' – 0.3/1.3], which is incorrectly marked on the USGS topo maps as being farther north. Ultimately, you cross several more tributaries before beginning the climb up to Donohue Pass. A short distance north of the last crossing, there are campsites on a bench to the west of the trail.

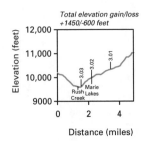

As you ascend, note the transition back to granitic substrate. However, in contrast to the granite of the southern Sierra, or that which you will shortly encounter in Yosemite, it has a darker color, as the granite's chemical composition changes near the boundary with the metamorphic rocks. Shortly, you reach the junction with the Marie Lakes Trail [10,040' – 0.9/2.2], where there are a couple of campsites, and you reach the roaring torrent of Rush Creek. A log bridge allows you to cross the flow safely. Climbing higher, you begin to exit forest cover, entering a landscape of wet meadows and small, drier hummocks. As the marshy, vegetated ground is mostly too wet and fragile for camping, only these whitebark-pine-speckled knobs offer dry, legal, and certainly worthwhile campsites—seek out sandy, previously used sites. As you climb ever higher, endless small creek crossings may slow your progress in early season. Even later in the year, the abundant heath vegetation is an indication of just how wet this area is: Dwarf bilberry, white heather, red heather, and bog kalmia are all common here, as are arctic willows. Look up from your feet as well and enjoy the broader view: an alpine, granite basin with abundant glacial erratics—large boulders scattered across the landscape where they were "dumped" by a glacier. Before long, you are following the final switchbacks up to the summit of tarn-dotted Donohue Pass [11,060' – 2.7/4.9], delineating the boundary between Yosemite National Park and Ansel Adams Wilderness. If you wish to climb still higher, a side trip up Donohue Peak is recommended (see Appendix E). Looking back, you can see Mammoth Mountain and the Mammoth Crest, country you have traversed over the past days.

Location	Elevation	Distance from Previous Point	Cumulative Distance	UTM Coordinates
Island Pass	10,205	—	0	11S 306699E 4178705N
Davis Lakes junction	9680	1.0	1.0	11S 305502E 4179278N
Rush Creek junction	9640	0.3	1.3	11S 305257E 4179482N
Marie Lakes junction	10,040	0.9	2.2	11S 304471E 4180124N
Donohue Pass	11,060	2.7	4.9	11S 302007E 4181469N

S–N
3

SECTION 2.

Donohue Pass to Tuolumne-Mariposa County Line—Tuolumne River

The descent begins on granite slabs and along sandy passageways, delineating fractures in the granite. Both red and white mountain heather form mats alongside rocks and near seasonal streams. The 13,114-foot summit of Mt. Lyell, the highest peak in Yosemite, looms to the southwest. The snowfield you see is the largest glacier visible from the JMT, and like most in the Sierra, one that has shrunk dramatically over the last century. Near the first ford of the Lyell Forks of the Tuolumne River are a few small sandy tent sites, used mainly by climbers headed toward Mt. Lyell. You traverse a small, dry, sandy knob and soon descend a steep slope crossed by numerous trickles and covered with lush vegetation. The grade eases in a wonderful timberline meadow that holds a small lake, across whose outlet you must make a chilly wade [10,185′ − 1.8/1.8]. On the northeast side of the crossing are a

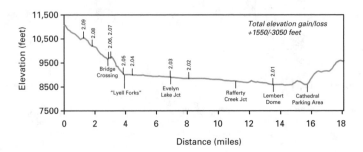

 SEE MAPS 11–12

few good campsites; many less ideal sites used by the latecomers are all near scattered stands of whitebark pines. Descending now through mixed hemlock and lodgepole forest, the JMT shortly crosses the Lyell Forks [9650' – 1.0/2.8] on a footbridge. Just beyond is a forested bench with many campsites. Following a brief uphill, the trail plunges down toward lovely, flat Lyell Canyon. You leave the last mountain hemlock stands behind and emerge onto a slope strewn with avalanche debris. One of the common shrubs on this disturbed slope is mountain red elderberry, distinguished by its large leaves, in clusters of seven; by midsummer, the berries are a favorite food source for wildlife.

At the base of the slope is an area where many river branches join called the "Lyell Forks" [9000' – 1.1/3.9]. This marks the beginning of a long, flat walk to Tuolumne Meadows. There are a few campsites just at

Location	Elevation	Distance from Previous Point	Cumulative Distance	UTM Coordinates
Donohue Pass	11,060	—	0	11S 302007E 4181469N
Wade across the Lyell Forks of the Tuolumne	10,185	1.8	1.8	11S 301333E 4182247N
Bridge across Lyell Forks of the Tuolumne	9650	1.0	2.8	11S 300860E 4183344N
Start of climb from Lyell Canyon (Lyell Forks)	9000	1.1	3.9	11S 300932E 4184713N
Evelyn Lake junction	8900	3.0	6.9	11S 299489E 4188820N
Rafferty Creek junction	8720	4.2	11.1	11S 295739E 4193385N
Eastern merge with alternate route	8670	0.7	11.8	11S 294824E 4193625N
Tuolumne High Sierra Camp junction	8680	0.6	12.4	11S 294688E 4194424N
Lembert Dome parking area	8585	1.1	13.5	11S 293124E 4194586N
Parsons Lodge junction	8565	0.7	14.2	11S 291899E 4194771N
Western merge with alternate route	8630	0.6	14.8	11S 291490E 4193887N
Cathedral Lakes parking area junction	8580	0.9	15.7	11S 290450E 4194131N
Mariposa-Tuolumne County line	9570	2.4	18.1	11S 287795E 4192140N

SEE MAP 12

the bottom of the switchbacks and others a short distance farther north. After a stretch through dry lodgepole forest, the trail trends toward the riverbank and often runs through the meadow lining the river. You get to enjoy this idyllic scene for the next many miles: The walls of Lyell Canyon rise steeply on either side; the unbelievably clear and often deep, aqua-green waters of the Lyell Forks meander down the middle of the canyon; if you are lucky, you will spot a belted kingfisher, with its shrill, cackling call, diving into the water to fish; and, of course, flower-filled meadows line the edges of the stream. Your only job is not to disturb the scene for the next party: Stay on the trail and do not trespass into the meadow each time the track becomes a bit deeper or muddier. Little elephant's heads, Sierra penstemon, alpine aster, alpine goldenrod, and club-moss ivesia all grace the meadow. With negligible elevation loss, you eventually reach Ireland Creek, which can easily be waded, or you can work your way across a series of logs to the west of the trail that are often half-submerged during high flow. Just beyond, you reach the junction with the trail to Ireland and Evelyn lakes [8900′ − 3.0/6.9]. To the northwest of this junction is the last major camping area before Tuolumne Meadows. A little downstream, at a position approximately marked by a large avalanche path visible on the east canyon wall, is the last legal camping before Tuolumne Meadows.

Where the river begins to bend westward, the trail diverges from the riverbank and you leave Lyell Canyon behind. Although you can't see it from the trail, you are still paralleling the Lyell Forks eastward, passing alternately through sections of lodgepole forest with little ground cover and through meadows, some marshy and others dominated by sedges. These areas are also a favorite haunt of the mule deer. The bucks are tame and sport large antlers in the sanctuary provided by the national park boundaries. Your next junction is with the Rafferty Creek Trail [8720′ − 4.2/11.1], which heads south to Vogelsang High Sierra Camp. Continuing through similar vegetation, you reach the next junction [8670′ − 0.7/11.8]. Here, the official JMT, and the route described here, heads north through Tuolumne Meadows, passing Lembert Dome and the historic Parsons Lodge. Although the official route is bit longer than the alternative, it is certainly the more scenic of the two options. However, many hikers opt to continue west at this trail junction, paralleling Hwy. 120, a more direct route to the Tuolumne Meadows campground and beyond. If you choose the latter, head due west, ignoring all junctions: past the first junction (turning north here leads you into the campground), past the Elizabeth Lake junction, continuing for approximately 2.3 miles through an open lodgepole forest

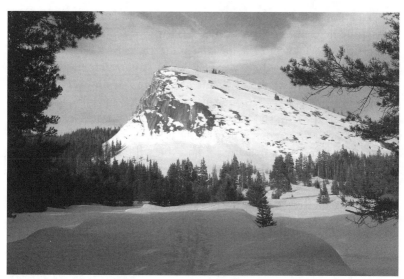

Lembert Dome in winter

until you rejoin the JMT at the second of two junctions leading to the visitor center.

Before we continue, a little Tuolumne Meadows orientation: Most Tuolumne Meadows amenities exist along the 1.5-mile, east-west Hwy. 120 corridor. From east to west, you will encounter the campground (the only legal camping until the lower Cathedral Lake), the grocery store, the Tuolumne Meadows Grill, a small mountaineering store, and a visitor center with an excellent bookstore and natural history displays. The Tuolumne Meadows campground has a section of walk-in campgrounds reserved for backpackers; these are due south of the Dana Campfire Circle and toward the eastern end of the campground. They cost $5 per person, and only a one-night stay is permitted. In addition, along a spur road, which you parallel while following the official JMT, is the Tuolumne Meadows Lodge, where showers are available during the middle of the day. Meals and lodging are also available, but must be reserved well in advance. Farther west along this road is the wilderness permit station.

Following the official JMT northward, you cross the Lyell Forks of the Tuolumne River on a pair of bridges, where you can gaze into the water at exquisitely carved granite—smooth slabs and deep holes, dangerous if the water is high and perfect for a cold dip later in the season. On the north side, still in dry lodgepole forest, the JMT curves west and north, leaving the Lyell Forks drainage and entering that of

SEE MAP 12

the Dana Fork. Over the next 3 miles, there are many trail junctions—keep your map out and eyes open. You first reach a junction with a trail headed northeast to Gaylor Lakes, shortly cross the Dana Fork on a footbridge, and immediately pass a signed spur trail to the Tuolumne Meadows Lodge (also known as the Tuolumne Meadows High Sierra Camp; 8680' – 0.6/12.4). Curving away from the Dana Fork, your route now parallels the spur road described before, first passing a large backpacker's parking lot, then emerging in a small meadow, and shortly reaching another large parking lot and the wilderness permit station. Here, rangers can both dispense wilderness permits and answer questions you pose regarding conditions. But please note that they are permitted only to dispense the most recent, factual information available to them; they cannot offer advice. This is often a source of frustration to both them and hikers. Leaving the wilderness permit station, you pick up a wide, dirt track that leads to the highway. Crossing Hwy. 120, you enter the Lembert Dome parking lot [8585' – 1.1/13.5], which provides a great view up the steep, granite face of Lembert Dome. The summit of Lembert Dome provides a 360-degree vista of the Tuolumne Meadows area; if you have a few hours, follow the trail northeast from the parking lot (see Appendix E).

The JMT follows the dirt road that trends west out of the Lembert Dome parking lot, the original route of Hwy. 120. Following it, you first pass a spur road to the local stables, then circumvent a gate that bars vehicular traffic, and shortly enter the meadow. Along this stretch, take your time to read the informative signs along the road, describing both the human and natural history of the area. Your path first takes you to the Soda Springs, where early tourists came to sample the soda water and relax. This was one of John Muir's favorite "hangouts" in Tuolumne, and where he conceived the idea of establishing Yosemite National Park. Just beyond, the ever-present metal trail signs point you south, across the Tuolumne River, but before you follow it, take a detour west up a small knob to Parsons Lodge and McCauley Cabin [8565' – 0.7/14.2]. The Sierra Club built Parsons Lodge as a mountain meeting room in 1915, and today it is filled with written and photographic tales of historical Tuolumne.

Now follow the JMT south, crossing the Tuolumne River on a footbridge. As you cross the flower-filled meadows, take note of the young lodgepole pines encroaching on the meadows. Researchers have several hypotheses for their relentless invasion, but they have not yet reached a consensus on the cause. This stretch of trail is also a good place to enjoy the landscape of nearby peaks and domes: To the south are Unicorn

SEE MAP 12

and Cathedral Range peaks and to the east are two large, red, rounded peaks, Mt. Dana and Mt. Gibbs. Pothole Dome, to the west, and Lembert Dome are good examples of roches moutonées. These domes, unlike some in Yosemite Valley, formed as a glacier flowed up and over their tops. The ascending side is smooth and gentle, while the glacier plucked large chunks of rock on the downhill side, creating a jagged, steep topography. On the south side of the meadow, you again cross Hwy. 120, pass a junction with a spur trail to the visitor center, and reach a T-junction where the trail paralleling the south side of the highway again merges with the official JMT route [8630' – 0.6/14.8]. Heading west (right), the JMT continues through open lodgepole forest, crosses Budd Creek on a footbridge, and reaches a junction where a large map of the area is posted [8580' – 0.9/15.7]. Turning right would take you to the Cathedral Lakes parking area, while the JMT turns left (south), toward the Cathedral Lakes. As you now leave Tuolumne Meadows behind, you no longer have to worry about heading the correct direction at the junctions you had been encountering every few minutes, and you can once again focus on the beautiful scenery.

You now ascend, still in dry, lodgepole-dominated forest, beneath which grow only a few alpine sticky currants and red heather. After some distance, the slope lessens, mountain hemlocks become more prevalent, and the ground becomes marshier; dwarf bilberry, western blueberry, and little elephant's heads are all present here. After some distance, you cross an avalanche zone with stunted trees and a view northwest to Fairview Dome. Climbing again, you are now in a forest dominated by mountain hemlock mixed with occasional western white pines. En route, you cross a small stream and later reach the robust spring that is its source. Before long, the ground again dries, the slope lessens, the herbaceous understory disappears, and lodegepole pines come to dominate. Shortly, you reach a seemingly un-noteworthy saddle, but this pass is the divide between the Tuolumne and Merced river drainages [9570' – 2.4/18.1]. There is no marker indicating when you cross the drainage divide, and it is difficult to decide when the grade becomes "downhill," but the results farther downstream couldn't be more dramatic: Water to the north flows down the Tuolumne River to Hetch Hetchy Reservoir and the plumbing of San Francisco, while water flowing into the Cathedral Lakes drains into Tenaya Lake and then down Tenaya Canyon to Yosemite Valley and the Merced River.

SECTION 1.

Tuolumne-Mariposa County Line to Happy Isles—Merced River

As you continue along the sandy shoulder, look over at Cathedral Peak, the steep granite spire to the east. This magnificent peak was first climbed by John Muir in 1869, via the slabs on the west face, the route at which you are gazing. Notice that the lower reaches are smooth and steep, having been rolled over by glaciers, while its summit is a jagged spire of jointed rock. Over the coming miles, you will pass many other peaks that share this profile. Entering denser forest again, you pass many small seeps and long stretches where the ground cover is dominated by dwarf bilberry, before reaching the junction with a lateral trail to the lower Cathedral Lake [9425' – 0.5/0.5], where you can find camping. Campfires are prohibited both here and at the upper Cathedral Lake, up ahead. You now climb gently through mixed lodgepole

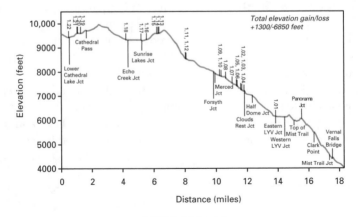

SEE MAP 12

and hemlock forest, entering a more open landscape as you approach the upper Cathedral Lake. The lake is nestled in a large meadow and is surrounded by the steep lower walls of Tresidder Peak and the Echo Peaks. A handful of campsites can be found in trees at the northern end of the lake and to the east of the trail in sandy patches. The trail crosses the often wet meadow before resuming its gradual climb to the broad saddle called Cathedral Pass [9700' – 1.1/1.6]. Here, alongside boulders, you will also be greeted by large masses of mountain pride penstemon. Continuing a climbing traverse across the east slope of Tresidder Peak, you approach a higher saddle—an excellent place to stop and enjoy the

Location	Elevation	Distance from Previous Point	Cumulative Distance	UTM Coordinates
Mariposa-Tuolumne County line	9570	—	0	11S 287795E 4192140N
Lower Cathedral Lake junction	9425	0.5	0.5	11S 287610E 4191528N
Cathedral Pass	9700	1.1	1.6	11S 287535E 4190040N
Echo Creek junction	9320	2.7	4.3	11S 286133E 4186544N
Sunrise Lakes junction	9320	0.9	5.2	11S 285841E 4185488N
Forsyth Trail junction	8010	4.6	9.8	11S 281726E 4181593N
Merced Lake junction	7960	0.1	9.9	11S 281692E 4181495N
Clouds Rest junction	7190	1.9	11.8	11S 279498E 4180201N
Half Dome junction	7015	0.5	12.3	11S 278771E 4180309N
Northeastern Little Yosemite Valley junction	6140	1.5	13.8	11S 278453E 4179139N
Western Little Yosemite Valley junction	6100	0.6	14.4	11S 277749E 4178733N
Nevada Fall junction	5980	0.6	15.0	11S 277073E 4178263N
Panorama Trail junction	6040	0.5	15.5	11S 276617E 4177802N
Clark Point junction	5480	0.8	16.3	11S 275787E 4178164N
Mist Trail junction	4600	1.0	17.3	11S 275458E 4178298N
Base of Vernal Fall	4390	0.2	17.5	11S 275238E 4178312N
Happy Isles	4035	0.8	18.3	11S 274640E 4178853N

SEE MAP 12

view of the Cathedral Range: the milelong, knife-edge Matthes Crest to your east, the Echo Peaks and Cathedral Peak to the northeast, and Columbia Finger and Tresidder Peak to the northwest. These are all spires of rock that once arose above the surrounding ice fields.

Leaving Tresidder Peak behind, you now descend more steeply through open lodgepole forest. Passing around Columbia Finger, you shortly reach Long Meadow. The notably steep north face of Columbia Finger certainly looks intimidating, and summiting it even via its easier west face requires a bit of scrambling, but there is an excellent view from its summit (see Appendix E). As you proceed southward, the upper stretches of Long Meadow transition to a forest, you pass a small campsite west of the trail, pass the Echo Creek Trail junction [9320′ − 2.7/4.3], and then re-emerge into the meadow. Continuing along the sandy western edge of Long Meadow, you enjoy the view south to the Clark Range and southeast to Mt. Florence, and then approach a point where the meadow bends to the right. Just beyond is the spur trail to the Sunrise High Sierra Camp; except for a few snacks, the camp has supplies only for its guests, who have reserved by lottery months in advance. A few more steps bring you to the junction with the trail to Sunrise Lakes and Clouds Rest [9320′ − 0.9/5.2]. Many campsites, bear boxes, and a pit toilet can be found a short distance up this trail.

The trail now contours around Sunrise Mountain, with only gentle changes in elevation. En route, you cross one small tributary where there is a small campsite among mountain hemlocks—your last chance to enjoy these wonderful trees. After you roll over the next sandy ridge, you descend to a meadow, alongside which there are several campsites. Alpine prickly currant, spreading phlox, and pussypaws are common here. Climbing again, the trail levels off on another large, sandy flat with scattered lodgepole pines. It might be difficult to believe that you have just completed your last climb of the JMT. As you descend toward Sunrise Creek, you leave behind the lodgepole forests that have accompanied you on so much of your walk. Indeed, western juniper and Jeffrey pines soon appear on the dry, south-facing slopes, and, lower still, western white pines and then red fir become the dominant species.

A few flat areas near your first crossing of Sunrise Creek provide good campsites in the dry, bare, red fir forest. Diverging again from Sunrise Creek, the JMT crosses over open flats, intersects the Forsyth Trail [8010′ − 4.6/9.8], and almost immediately thereafter meets the junction with a trail to Merced Lake [7960′ − 0.1/9.9]. Soon, alongside a tributary of Sunrise Creek, you will find several more pleasant campsites. As you descend, the red fir are slowly replaced by the longer-needled white fir. Creeping snowberry is a common ground cover throughout these dry forests. Pygmy nuthatches, a smaller version of the red-breasted nuthatch, and blue grouse are likely seen here. Just after you cross Sunrise Creek, a collection of use trails leads north to campsites atop a small knob dotted with Jeffrey pines. These campsites provide delightful views toward Half Dome and Mt. Starr King, a dome south of the Merced River canyon. The JMT continues down the north bank of Sunrise Creek, passing occasional campsites. In places, you can enjoy western azaleas lining the stream; in early season, they are thickly covered in aromatic white flowers. As you descend one small set of switchbacks, note the large, flat camping area alongside Sunrise Creek and beneath towering trees—an often crowded, but beautiful spot. Minutes further down the trail, you cross a small tributary and find additional small campsites surrounding the Clouds Rest Trail junction [7190' – 1.9/11.8]. The summit of Clouds Rest, accessible by trail, is a worthwhile detour, with outstanding views of Yosemite Valley, Half Dome, and the Yosemite high country (see Appendix E).

Descending ever lower, you are now entering new vegetation zones. In addition to Jeffrey pines, a few sugar pines, with enormous, elongate cones, grace the forest. Incense cedars, with shaggy red bark and minute, scaly leaves, grow in flats. California black oak are large, deciduous trees identified by their large, lobed leaves. The next stretch of trail is across a dry slope with dense scrub cover and only scattered trees: The underlying slabs are close to the surface, and in many places, the soil is insufficiently deep for trees. Here are dense stands of canyon live oak, a shrub with small, leathery leaves. In half a mile, the JMT meets the lateral to Half Dome [7015' – 0.5/12.3], an incredible 4-mile round trip that shouldn't be missed (see Appendix E).

Your descent continues through a predominately white fir forest that is interspersed with sugar pines and Jeffrey pines. Elsewhere are flat stretches lined by magnificent incense cedars. In a few places, the forest canopy opens, and you can glance northwest to Half Dome. Before long, you reach a junction [6140' – 1.5/13.8], where the JMT takes a left turn toward the Little Yosemite Valley camping area and the Merced River. To take a shortcut, continue straight ahead; the two traits merge a short distance to the west. The camping area, the last legal campsites before Yosemite Valley, has toilets and bear boxes. Within five minutes, you reach a T-junction and turn right (west), paralleling the unseen Merced River downstream through dense forest. In early season, you may see the peculiar red snowplant that is non-photosynthetic and obtains nutrients from nearby tree roots. Near where your

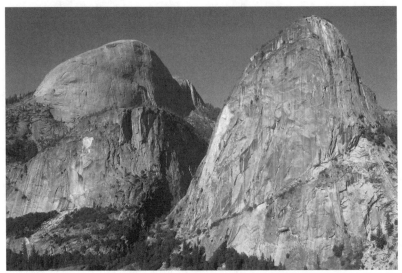

Half Dome (upper left), Mt. Broderick (lower left), and Liberty Cap

path intersects the Merced River, the shortcut merges with the JMT [6100' – 0.6/14.4], and your flat, westward walk continues beside a stream bank densely covered with western azaleas. Following a slight rise, you find yourself descending sandy, rocky switchbacks, on which vegetation includes canyon live oak; Fremont silktassel, with long, dangling tassels of flowers; black oak; and occasionally a towering Jeffrey or sugar pine. The zigzags end atop the Mist Trail, near some restrooms [5980' – 0.6/15.0].

From this point, you can continue down the more graded JMT or, if your knees are feeling strong, take the steeper Mist Trail, whose route more closely follows the steep river channel, often on steep stairs. Assuming you wish to follow the official route, continue south along the top of the escarpment. Climbing briefly, you emerge onto open slabs beside the Merced River and follow a line of rocks westward to the top of Nevada Fall. A spur trail leads to a fenced vista point, and the JMT crosses a sturdy footbridge over the often raging waters. Shortly, you pass a signed junction with the Panorama Trail [6040' – 0.5/15.5] and begin a panoramic traverse along a trail blasted into the cliff. Stop regularly and enjoy the vista, which is especially spectacular near the west end of the walled-in traverse. To the northeast is the rounded backside of Half Dome, and to the east, Nevada Fall drops 594 feet. Mt. Broderick and Liberty Cap are the two prominent domes behind Nevada Fall. While these domes were glaciated, their rounded tops actually exist due

SEE MAP 13

to exfoliation of their constituent granite—imagine the peeling-off layers of an onion. In comparison, many of the domes dotting Tuolumne Meadows still have smoother, more polished summits. Most of the flowers here bloom before the JMT hikers pass by, but damp sections of this trail are still colorful in late season: California fuchsias is a low-growing shrub with bright red, tubular flowers, and grass-of-Parnassus has creamy white, five-petal flowers on tall stems.

After descending yet more switchbacks, you shortly reach the Clark Point junction [5480' – 0.8/16.3], your last chance to take in the view of the waterfalls and the surrounding canyon. If you descend the trail north from Clark Point, you will intersect the Mist Trail near the top of Vernal Fall, while the JMT continues down the left-hand trail fork. Ahead of you now is a long stretch of switchbacks, seemingly interminable, since your journey is almost over, and tough on your feet, since many were once paved. The tree species on this slope are mostly unique to this stretch of the JMT. Douglas fir is the main conifer species, while three broadleaf species are California black oak, big-leaf maples, and California bay-laurels, with long, skinny, leathery, and highly aromatic leaves. Steller's jays, a variety of woodpeckers, California ground squirrels, and western gray squirrels are all common along the trail. Where the grade lessens, you pass a signed horse trail coming in from the west, and just thereafter reach the junction with the base of the Mist Trail [4600' – 1.0/17.3]

Now just a mile from the trailhead, the ever-increasing number of dayhikers can be overwhelming. Paralleling the turbulent river's south bank, you continue a short distance downstream to a stout footbridge across the Merced River [4390' – 0.2/17.5]. Here are restrooms and a drinking fountain—refurbished with spouts for both drinking and filling water bottles. There is a superb view of Vernal Fall from the footbridge; be sure to pull out your camera. Across the bridge, the JMT turns west, curving around the base of Sierra Point, a popular vista point before a rockfall closed the trail many years ago. Descending the last stretch of asphalt-covered trail, you shortly find yourself in front of a large sign, proclaiming the end of the JMT. Congratulations! You do still have to continue a short distance north to a paved road and then west across the Merced River to the free shuttlebus stop [4035' – 0.8/18.3].

APPENDIX A.

Mileage Square

	Happy Isles	Half Dome junction	Mariposa-Tuolumne County line	Rafferty Creek junction	Donohue Pass	Island Pass	Northern Devils Postpile junction	Madera-Fresno County line	Tully Hole junction
Happy Isles	0.0								
Half Dome junction	6.0	0.0							
Mariposa-Tuolumne County line	18.3	12.3	0.0						
Rafferty Creek junction	25.3	19.3	7.0	0.0					
Donohue Pass	36.4	30.4	18.1	11.1	0.0				
Island Pass	41.3	35.3	23.0	16.0	4.9	0.0			
Northern Devils Postpile junction	56.3	50.3	38.0	31.0	19.9	15.0	0.0		
Madera-Fresno County line	63.8	57.8	45.5	38.5	27.4	22.5	7.5	0.0	
Tully Hole junction	76.6	70.6	58.3	51.3	40.2	35.3	20.3	12.8	0.0
Silver Pass	81.1	75.1	62.8	55.8	44.7	39.8	24.8	17.3	4.5
Lake Edison junction	87.6	81.6	69.3	62.3	51.2	46.3	31.3	23.8	11.0
Selden Pass	101.4	95.4	83.1	76.1	65.0	60.1	45.1	37.6	24.8
JMT southern cutoff	108.8	102.8	90.5	83.5	72.4	67.5	52.5	45.0	32.2
Muir Pass	127.9	121.9	109.6	102.6	91.5	86.6	71.6	64.1	51.3
Bishop Pass junction	135.7	129.7	117.4	110.4	99.3	94.4	79.4	71.9	59.1
Mather Pass	149.6	143.6	131.3	124.3	113.2	108.3	93.3	85.8	73.0
Pinchot Pass	159.4	153.4	141.1	134.1	123.0	118.1	103.1	95.6	82.8
Glen Pass	175.3	169.3	157.0	150.0	138.9	134.0	119.0	111.5	98.7
Kearsarge Pass junction	177.3	171.3	159.0	152.0	140.9	136.0	121.0	113.5	100.7
Forester Pass	187.1	181.1	168.8	161.8	150.7	145.8	130.8	123.3	110.5
PCT junction west of Crabtree Meadows	199.9	193.9	181.6	174.6	163.5	158.6	143.6	136.1	123.3
Mt. Whitney	208.2	202.2	189.9	182.9	171.8	166.9	151.9	144.4	131.6
Trail Crest	210.3	204.3	192.0	185.0	173.9	169.0	154.0	146.5	133.7
Whitney Portal	218.5	212.5	200.2	193.2	182.1	177.2	162.2	154.7	141.9

Silver Pass	Lake Edison junction	Selden Pass	JMT southern cutoff	Muir Pass	Bishop Pass junction	Mather Pass	Pinchot Pass	Glen Pass	Kearsarge Pass junction	Forester Pass	PCT junction west of Crabtree Meadows	Mt. Whitney	Trail Crest	Whitney Portal
0.0														
6.5	0.0													
20.3	13.8	0.0												
27.7	21.2	7.4	0.0											
46.8	40.3	26.5	19.1	0.0										
54.6	48.1	34.3	26.9	7.8	0.0									
68.5	62.0	48.2	40.8	21.7	13.9	0.0								
78.3	71.8	58.0	50.6	31.5	23.7	9.8	0.0							
94.2	87.7	73.9	66.5	47.4	39.6	25.7	15.9	0.0						
96.2	89.7	75.9	68.5	49.4	41.6	27.7	17.9	2.0	0.0					
106.0	99.5	85.7	78.3	59.2	51.4	37.5	27.7	11.8	9.8	0.0				
118.8	112.3	98.5	91.1	72.0	64.2	50.3	40.5	24.6	22.6	12.8	0.0			
127.1	120.6	106.8	99.4	80.3	72.5	58.6	48.8	32.9	30.9	21.1	8.3	0.0		
129.2	122.7	108.9	101.5	82.4	74.6	60.7	50.9	35.0	33.0	23.2	10.4	2.1	0.0	
137.4	130.9	117.1	109.7	90.6	82.8	68.9	59.1	43.2	41.2	31.4	18.6	10.3	8.2	0.0

APPENDIX B.

JMT Lateral Trails
and Food Resupply Options

You may need to use JMT lateral trails for a variety of reasons—to resupply on food, because you are hiking only part of the trail, or to bail out if the weather turns bad or a member of your party is sick or injured. This appendix includes information on the lateral trails, towns near the JMT, places to mail resupply packages, and stock resupply.

While there are many lateral trails from which you can exit the JMT, most hikers pick up packages at some of the following locations: Tuolumne Meadows Post Office, Reds Meadow Resort near Devils Postpile, Vermilion Valley Resort (via the Lake Edison Trail), Muir Trail Ranch (via the Florence Lake Trail), Bishop Post Office (via the Bishop Pass Trail), and the Independence Post Office (via the Kearsarge Pass Trail). If you plan to buy food as you go, Yosemite Valley, Tuolumne Meadows, Mammoth Lakes, and Bishop all have shops that sell a variety of backpacking food. The stores at Reds Meadow Resort and Vermilion Valley Resort are also adequate.

In general, exiting the JMT becomes more difficult the farther south you are: There are many relatively easy options in the northern third of the trail, a few long, but well-graded and well-maintained options in the middle third of the trail (e.g. Mono Pass, Piute Pass, and Bishop Pass), and only one well-maintained option from Bishop Pass south (Kearsarge Pass). Toward the south, some of the trails heading out to the west side are easier and shorter, because you don't have to cross the crest. But keep in mind that the western trailheads are very isolated, and finding a ride back to a population center or your car may prove very difficult.

JMT Lateral Trails

This section details your on/off options from north to south along the JMT. It does not, however, include cross-country routes (e.g. Italy Pass) or junctions whose routes to the nearest trailhead are more than

20 miles in length (e.g. Goddard Canyon, the High Sierra Trail). Most of the route and trailhead information is drawn from other Wilderness Press books, including *Sierra North, Sierra South, Kings Canyon National Park,* and *Sequoia National Park.* If you know in advance that you will be using one of the JMT lateral trails for a food resupply or because you are section-hiking, consult those volumes for greater detail about these routes.

The following details on lateral trails tell you:

- The trail junction's location (UTM coordinates and elevation) and distance from the terminuses of the JMT: Happy Isles in Yosemite Valley to the north (YV) and Whitney Portal in the south (WP).
- Topos covering the route: "USGS" indicates a USGS 7.5-minute topo, and "TH" indicates a Tom Harrison map.
- Agency in whose jurisdiction the trailhead is and the trailhead for which you need to obtain a permit. Abbreviations: YNP = Yosemite National Park; SiNF = Sierra National Forest; INF = Inyo National Forest; SEKI = Sequoia and Kings Canyon national parks.
- Hikes are described from the JMT out to a trailhead.
- Driving directions to the trailhead are described from the nearest town to the trailhead.

Tuolumne Meadows, Toward Cathedral Lakes

Access to West Side: Tuolumne Meadows at Cathedral Lakes Trailhead

Location: 11S 290450E 4194131N; 8580′

Distance from Endpoints: 20.7 miles from YV; 197.8 miles from WP

Maps: USGS *Tenaya Lake, Tioga Pass, Vogelsang Peak;* TH *Yosemite High Country*

Permits: YNP: Cathedral Lakes Trailhead

The Hike: 0.1 mile; head a short distance north from the Cathedral Lakes Trailhead

Trailhead Amenities: Visitor center, store, small cafe, campground, and (during midday) showers at the lodge

Getting to the Trailhead: The Cathedral Lakes Trailhead, near the western end of Tuolumne Meadows, is 8.3 miles southwest of Tioga Pass on Hwy. 120.

Tuolumne Meadows, South to Lyell Canyon

Access to West Side: Tuolumne Meadows at wilderness permit parking area

Location: 11S 293773E 4194515N; 8650′

Distance from Endpoints: 23.4 miles from YV; 195.1 mile from WP

Maps: USGS *Tenaya Lake, Tioga Pass, Vogelsang Peak*; TH *Yosemite High Country*

Permits: YNP: Lyell Canyon Trailhead, Upper Lyell Trailhead

The Hike: None

Trailhead Amenities: Visitor center, store, small cafe, campground, and (during midday) showers at the lodge

Getting to the Trailhead: On Hwy. 120, just east of the Lembert Dome parking lot and 6.5 miles southwest of Tioga Pass is a signed turnoff for Tuolumne Lodge. Turn right here and go a short way down the turnoff, then take a hard right onto a spur and into the backpacker's parking lot. Additional parking is available a short distance east along the road toward the Tuolumne Lodge. The JMT passes through the meadow just south of the road.

Rush Creek Trail

Access to East Side: June Lake

Location: 11S 305257E 4179482N; 9640'

Distance from Endpoints: 40 miles from YV; 178.5 miles from WP

Maps: USGS *Mt. Ritter, Koip Peak*; TH *Mammoth High Country*

Permits: INF: Rush Creek Trailhead

The Hike: 10.3 miles (allow one or two days); go east on Rush Creek Trail to Silver Lake on State Route 158. No passes to cross; campsites along the way.

Trailhead Amenities: Toilets, campground, and Silver Lake Resort

Getting to the Trailhead: From the southern junction of Hwy. 395 and State Route 158, drive southwest for 7.3 miles through June Lake village, past June Mountain Ski Area, and just past Silver Lake Resort, to a large parking lot west of the road.

Shadow Lake Trail to Agnew Meadows

Access to East Side: Mammoth Lakes

Location: 11S 311695E 4173764N; 8760'

Distance from Endpoints: 48.6 miles from YV; 169.9 miles from WP

Maps: USGS *Mt. Ritter, Mammoth Mtn.*; TH *Mammoth High Country*

Permits: INF: Shadow Lake Trailhead

The Hike: 3.5 miles; go east past Shadow Lake to Agnew Meadows, then walk a quarter mile on a dirt spur road to find Devils Postpile Road. Take the seasonal shuttlebus to Mammoth Mountain Ski Area/Bike Park.

Trailhead Amenities: Toilets

Getting to the Trailhead: At the junction of Hwy. 395 and State Route 203, drive west for 3.8 miles through the town of Mammoth Lakes to the intersection where 203 turns right, toward Mammoth Mountain

Ski Area and Devils Postpile. Turn right and drive 4.2 miles to the main Mammoth Mountain Ski Area. Between 7 a.m. and 7:30 p.m. from mid-June through September, you are obliged to park here and take a shuttlebus into the postpile area. Before 7 a.m. and after 7:30 p.m., you may drive your own car, in which case you continue another 4.1 miles up and over Minaret Summit and down to the Agnew Meadows Trailhead, located at the first hairpin turn. You can park in either of the two lots; the trailhead is on the south side of the first lot. Whether traveling by shuttlebus or private vehicle, there is a $7 per person use fee. See www.nps.gov/depo for additional information.

Devils Postpile

Access to East Side: Mammoth Lakes
Location: 11S 315747E 4166939N; 7685'
Distance from Endpoints: 56.3 miles from YV; 162.2 miles from WP
Maps: USGS *Mammoth Mtn.*; TH *Mammoth High Country*
Permits: INF: JMT/PCT South Trailhead if heading south; JMT/PCT North Trailhead if heading north
The Hike: 0.7 mile; go southeast to the Middle Fork of San Joaquin River opposite Devils Postpile. Cross the bridge over the river, and at the next junction, go left a short distance to the visitor center and a stop for seasonal shuttlebus service to Mammoth Mountain Ski Area.
Trailhead Amenities: Toilets, water, campground, visitor center, and several nearby campgrounds.
Getting to the Trailhead: Follow the directions to Agnew Meadows (page 224) as far as the hairpin turn; don't turn here, but continue on the paved road to the signed turnoff for Devils Postpile. The distance from the Mammoth Mountain Ski Area parking lot is 8.1 miles.

Reds Meadow Resort

Access to East Side: Mammoth Lakes, Reds Meadow Resort
Location: 11S 316900E 4164357N; 7715'
Distance from Endpoints: 58.7 miles from YV; 159.8 miles from WP
Maps: USGS *Crystal Crag*; TH *Mammoth High Country*
Permits: INF: JMT/PCT South Trailhead if heading south; JMT/PCT North Trailhead if heading north
The Hike: 0.3 mile; go north to the Reds Meadow Resort and a stop for seasonal shuttlebus service to Mammoth Mountain Ski Area.
Trailhead Amenities: Toilet, water, Reds Meadow Resort (seasonal lodging, cafe, store), and other campgrounds nearby, including Reds Meadow Campground (hot-spring-fed showers)
Getting to the Trailhead: Follow the directions on page 224 to Agnew Meadows as far as the hairpin turn; don't turn here. Continue on the paved road to the signed turnoff for Devils Postpile. At this junction,

continue on the road to a Y-junction, and turn left on a paved road to Reds Meadow Resort. The right turn leads down a dirt road to a parking lot for Rainbow Falls. The total distance from the Mammoth Mountain Ski Area parking lot is 9.6 miles.

Mammoth Pass Trail from Upper Crater Meadow

Access to East Side: Mammoth Lakes

Location: 11S 319252E 4161498N; 8915'. Note that there are several other nearby trail junctions with trails heading over Mammoth Pass. This is the most clearly signposted and the best-used trail.

Distance from Endpoints: 62.7 miles from YV; 155.8 miles from WP

Maps: USGS *Crystal Crag*; TH *Mammoth High Country*

Permits: INF: Red Cones Trailhead

The Hike: 3 miles; go north on rolling terrain to meet the trail from lower Crater Meadow in 1.2 miles. Continue north, then east, over forested Mammoth Pass (9350'), to McCloud Lake, near the east end of which you find a junction with a trail going northwest. You go ahead, east and northeast, to the trailhead at Horseshoe Lake.

Trailhead Amenities: Toilets. You are in a lakes basin southwest of Mammoth Lakes, and there are campgrounds, lodgings, and a few stores widely scattered along the roads through the basin.

Getting to the Trailhead: At the junction of Hwy. 395 and State Route 203, drive west for 3.8 miles through the town of Mammoth Lakes to the intersection where 203 turns right, toward Mammoth Mountain Ski Resort and Devils Postpile. Continue straight ahead, now on the Lake Mary Road, and follow it past a turnoff to Twin Lakes and the Mammoth Pack Station. At a T-junction, head straight ahead around Lake Mary's north shore and head toward Lake Mamie and Horseshoe Lake. Continue straight all the way to the road's end at Horseshoe Lake, about 5.7 miles past the junction to the Mammoth Mountain Ski Area.

Duck Pass Trail

Access to East Side: Mammoth Lakes

Location: 11S 326105E 4156217N; 10,170'

Distance from Endpoints: 70.3 miles from YV; 148.2 miles from WP

Maps: USGS *Bloody Mtn.*; TH *Mammoth High Country*

Permits: INF: Duck Lake Trailhead

The Hike: 6 miles (allow one day); go over Duck Pass (10,797'; snow possible on north side) to Coldwater Canyon Trailhead. There are campsites along the way; no camping within 300 feet of Duck Lake's outlet.

Trailhead Amenities: Toilets, water, campground. You are in a lakes basin southwest of Mammoth Lakes, and there are campgrounds, lodgings, and a few stores widely scattered along the roads through the basin.

Getting to the Trailhead: At the junction of Hwy. 395 and State Route 203, drive west for 3.8 miles through the town of Mammoth Lakes to the intersection where 203 turns right, toward Mammoth Mountain Ski Area and Devils Postpile. Continue straight ahead, now on the Lake Mary Road, and follow it past a turnoff to Twin Lakes and the Mammoth Pack Station. At a T-junction, turn left to skirt Lake Mary's eastern shore. At a second T-junction, past Pine City Campground, turn left into Coldwater Campground and follow signs to a large parking lot at the top of Coldwater Campground, 5.2 miles past the junction to the Mammoth Mountain Ski Area. The Duck Pass Trail begins behind the toilets. Do not take the spur trail that immediately heads up and left toward Emerald Lake.

McGee Pass Trail

Access to East Side: Crowley Lake, 10 miles south of Mammoth Lakes on Hwy. 395

Location: 11S 329943E 4152061N; 9520′

Distance from Endpoints: 76.6 miles from YV; 141.9 miles from WP

Maps: USGS *Bloody Mtn.*, *Graveyard Peak*, *Mt. Abbott*, *Convict Lake*; TH *Mammoth High Country*, *Mono Divide High Country*

Permits: INF: McGee Creek Trailhead

The Hike: 15.5 miles (allow one to two days); head up Fish Creek and over rugged McGee Pass (11,909′; snow likely on east side) to McGee Creek Trailhead. There are campsites along the way.

Trailhead Amenities: Toilet, nearby campground, and pack station down the road

Getting to the Trailhead: From Hwy. 395 between Bishop and Mammoth Lakes, turn southwest on signed McGee Canyon Road and follow it 3.2 miles past McGee Pack Station to a roadend parking loop.

Mono Pass Trail

Access to East Side: Toms Place, 24 miles north of Bishop; 15 miles south of Mammoth Lakes from Hwy. 395

Location: 11S 331029E 4143228N; 8350′

Distance from Endpoints: 86.2 miles from YV; 132.3 miles from WP

Maps: USGS *Graveyard Peak*, *Mt. Abbot*, *Mt. Morgan*; TH *Mono Divide High Country*

Permits: INF: Mono Pass Trailhead

The Hike: 15.1 miles (allow one to two days); go east up Mono Creek and over Mono Pass (12,000′) to Mosquito Flat Trailhead. There are campsites along the way.

Trailhead Amenities: Toilets and, down Rock Creek Road, camp-grounds, lodging, cafes, and stores

Getting to the Trailhead: From Hwy. 395 at Toms Place, turn west on Rock Creek Road and follow the road past Rock Creek Lake. Beyond the turnoff for the lake, the road shortly becomes one lane. Continue all the way to the roadend parking lot, 9.2 miles from Hwy. 395.

Lake Edison Trail   559 841 -3404

Access to West Side: Lake Thomas Edison, Vermilion Valley Resort, Mono Hot Springs

Location: 11S 329758E 4142189N; 7900'

Distance from Endpoints: 87.6 miles from YV; 130.9 miles from WP

Maps: USGS *Graveyard Peak, Sharktooth Peak;* TH *Mono Divide High Country*

Permits: Sierra NF: Mono Creek Trailhead

The Hike: 1 mile to ferry or 4.5 miles to trailhead; go southwest to a junction with a spur trail to a landing for twice-daily ferry service (seasonal; fee) across Lake Edison to Vermilion Valley Resort at the lake's west end. Alternatively, continue around the northern shore of Lake Edison to the trailhead at Vermilion Campground.

Trailhead Amenities: Campground, water, and toilets

Getting to the Trailhead: Take State Route 168 through Clovis and up into the foothills, through the community of Shaver Lake. Continue straight ahead at a turnoff to Huntington Lake and the community of Lakeshore, on what is now Kaiser Pass Road. The road shortly becomes narrow and twisting. At Kaiser Pass, it becomes even more narrow and twisting before descending past the High Sierra ranger station to a Y-junction. A left turn here heads to Mono Hot Springs Resort, Lake Edison, and Vermilion Valley Resort, and a right turn goes to Florence Lake. Turn left once you are past the turnoffs to Mono Hot Springs and Vermilion Valley resorts, as the road turns to dirt. Pass the first turnoff for Vermilion Campground, pass the pack station turnoff, and follow the road through the campground to the farthest end of the easternmost campground loop, where there's a parking area bounded by huge logs, more than 89 miles from Clovis.

Bear Ridge Trail

Access to West Side: Lake Thomas Edison

Location: 11S 330945E 4138822N; 9880'

Distance from Endpoints: 92.2 miles from YV; 126.3 miles from WP

Maps: USGS *Florence Lake, Graveyard Peak;* TH *Mono Divide High Country*

Permits: Sierra NF: Bear Ridge Trailhead

The Hike: 5 miles; go west down to the Bear Ridge parking area at the eastern edge of the Lake Thomas Edison dam.

Trailhead Amenities: Toilets and, nearby, Vermilion Valley Resort and several campgrounds

Getting to the Trailhead: Refer to the driving directions to Lake Edison on page 228. However, just as you approach the dam across Lake Edison, turn right into a parking lot.

Bear Creek Trail

Access to West Side: Lake Thomas Edison, Mono Hot Springs
Location: 11S 332858E 4137219N; 8970'
Distance from Endpoints: 94.3 miles from YV; 124.2 miles from WP
Maps: USGS *Florence Lake, Mt. Givens*; TH *Mono Divide High Country*
Permits: Sierra NF: Bear Diversion Trailhead
The Hike: 9 miles (allow for one day); go southwest down Bear Creek. The last 2.5 miles from Bear Diversion Dam is on an OHV road. There are campsites along the way.

Trailhead Amenities: Nearby are several campgrounds, Mono Hot Springs Resort, and a post office. Head 1 mile south on the Kaiser Pass Road, and then turn right, to the west, and head a short distance down a spur road signed for Mono Hot Springs.

Getting to this Trailhead: Refer to the driving directions to Lake Edison on page 228. Turn left at the Y-junction, as for Lake Edison, but in 2.5 miles, find the Bear Diversion Dam road junction (with an OHV route) on your right. Passenger cars can't go beyond here; the OHV route goes 2.5 more miles to Bear Diversion Dam, and high-clearance 4WD vehicles may be able to make it.

Florence Lake Trail past Muir Trail Ranch

Access to West Side: Florence Lake, Muir Trail Ranch
Location: Northern JMT cutoff: 11S 334054E 4123186N; 8400'
Southern JMT cutoff: 11S 334959E 4121342N; 7880'
Junction between two JMT cutoffs: 11S 333529E 4122654N; 7800'
Distance from Endpoints: Northern JMT cutoff: 107.1 miles from YV; 111.4 miles from WP
Southern JMT cutoff: 108.8 miles from YV; 109.7 miles from WP
Maps: USGS *Florence Lake, Ward Mountain*; TH *Mono Divide High Country*
Permits: Sierra NF: Florence
The Hike: Variable, by destination. From the northern JMT cutoff, descend switchbacks for approximately 0.9 mile to the junction between the two JMT cutoffs. From the southern JMT cutoff, follow the nearly flat Florence Lake Trail along the South Fork of the San Joaquin River for 1.5 miles to the junction between the JMT cutoffs.

From this junction, continue 0.25 mile west to a well-marked junction for the Muir Trail Ranch, to which you can mail a food drop (see end of this appendix for details). If you follow the first turnoff to the Muir Trail Ranch, you will shortly reach a second junction: left to cross the San Joaquin River to Blayney Hot Springs (note that there is no bridge, and the river is dangerous to ford during heavy runoff), and right to the Muir Trail Ranch.

To reach Florence Lake, hike 5 more miles to a spur trail to the landing for a ferry service (seasonal; fee) across Florence Lake to the trailhead. Or, from the spur trail junction, continue an additional 5 miles around the lake to the trailhead. There are campsites along the way.

Trailhead Amenities: Toilets, water, and Florence Lake Store

Getting to the Trailhead: Follow the directions under the Lake Edison Trail (page 228) as far as the Y-junction, and turn right to Florence Lake. Follow this very poor, very narrow road to the roadend parking area, about 87 miles from Clovis.

Pine Creek Pass Trail and Piute Pass Trail

Access to East Side: Bishop

Location: 11S 337415E 4121216N; 8050'

Distance from Endpoints: 110.6 miles from YV; 107.9 miles from WP

Maps: USGS *Mt. Henry, Mt. Hilgard, Mt. Darwin, Mt. Tom;* TH *Mono Divide High Country*

Permits: INF: Pine Creek TH or Piute Pass TH

The Hike (via Pine Creek Pass): 17.6 miles (allow two to three days); go northeast about 4.6 miles to a junction at Hutchinson Meadow, passing few campsites. Follow the left-hand, northeastern trail through French Canyon over Pine Creek Pass (11,100') to Pine Creek Trailhead.

Trailhead Amenities: Toilets and pack station

Getting to the Trailhead: From Bishop, head north on Hwy. 395 for 10 miles to the signed road to Rovana. Follow this road 10 miles west to a signed parking area beside Pine Creek.

The Hike (via Piute Pass): 15.6 miles (allow two to three days); go northeast about 4.6 miles to a junction at Hutchinson Meadow, passing few campsites. Follow the right-hand, southeastern trail through Humphreys Basin over Piute Pass (11,423') to North Lake Campground.

Trailhead Amenities: Campground, toilets, water, and pack station

Getting to the Trailhead: From the junction of Hwy. 395 and State Route 168 (West Line Street) in Bishop, go southwest 18 miles. A mile after the town of Aspendell, turn right onto a dirt road to North Lake. Go 2 miles to a backpacker's parking area just beyond North Lake and next to the pack station. The trailhead is a half mile ahead, in the North Lake Campground (no parking).

Bishop Pass Trail

Access to East Side: Bishop
Location: 11S 358398E 4106234N; 8720′
Distance from Endpoints: 135.7 miles from YV; 82.8 miles from WP
Maps: USGS *North Palisade, Mt. Thompson*; TH *Kings Canyon High Country*
Permits: INF: Bishop Pass Trailhead
The Hike: 11.6 miles (allow for one to two days); go east on switchbacks out of the steep-walled Le Conte Canyon, through Dusy Basin, and over Bishop Pass (11,972′) to the South Lake Trailhead. There are campsites along the way.
At the Trailhead: Toilets and, nearby, pack station, campgrounds, and resorts
Getting to the Trailhead: From the junction of Hwy. 395 and State Route 168 (West Line Street) in Bishop, go southwest 15.5 miles to a fork. Turn left and go 7 more miles to parking at South Lake.

Taboose Pass Trail

Access to East Side: Hwy. 395, 12 miles south of Big Pine, 15 miles north of Independence
Location: 11S 371999E 4091458N; 10,780′
Distance from Endpoints: 156.3 miles from YV; 62.2 miles from WP
Maps: USGS *Mt. Pinchot, Aberdeen*; TH *Kings Canyon High Country*
Permits: INF: Taboose Pass Trailhead
The Hike: 10 miles (allow for one to two days); go over Taboose Pass (11,418′) to make a steep descent to Taboose Creek Roadend, passing only a few campsites along the way. This is a difficult trail.
Trailhead Amenities: None
Getting to the Trailhead: From Hwy. 395, 12 miles south of Big Pine or 15 miles north of Independence, turn west onto paved Taboose Creek Road. Go straight ahead at a four-way junction with Tinemaha Road. After 3.5 miles from Hwy. 395, head right at a Y, and continue another 2 miles to the trailhead. This is a very low-use trail, and finding a ride to Big Pine or Independence is likely to be difficult.

Sawmill Pass Trail

Access to East Side: Hwy. 395, 17.5 miles south of Big Pine, 9.5 miles north of Independence
Location: 11S 375312E 4084783N; 10,345′
Distance from Endpoints: 163.1 miles from YV; 55.4 miles from WP

Maps: USGS *Mt. Pinchot, Aberdeen;* TH *Kings Canyon High Country*
Permits: INF: Sawmill Pass Trailhead
The Hike: 12.5 miles (allow one to two days); go east on an unmaintained and, in sections, steep trail, into a lakes basin with few campsites. Then head over Sawmill Pass (11,347'), past the Sawmill Lakes (camping) and descend to the Sawmill Creek Roadend. Although the west side of the pass has been maintained recently, this is a difficult trail.
Trailhead Amenities: None
Getting to the Trailhead: From Hwy. 395, 17.5 miles south of Big Pine or 9.5 miles north of Independence, turn west onto the dirt Black Rock Springs Road. Go west 0.8 mile to a junction with Tinemaha Road. Turn right and continue for 1.2 miles. Then turn left onto Division Creek Road and follow it for 1.9 miles to the trailhead. This is a very low-use trail, and finding a ride to Big Pine or Independence is likely to be difficult.

Woods Creek Trail

Access to West Side: Roads End at Cedar Grove
Location: 11S 371810E 4081629N; 8592'
Distance from Endpoints: 166.6 miles from YV; 51.9 miles from WP
Maps: USGS *Mt. Clarence King, The Sphinx;* TH *Kings Canyon High Country*
Permits: SEKI: Wood's Creek Trail
The Hike: 13.5 miles (allow one to two days); go southwest through Paradise Valley to Roads End at Cedar Grove (5035') in Kings Canyon. There are campsites and bear boxes on the way; no camping below Paradise Valley.
Trailhead Amenities: Toilets, National Park Service ranger station and, nearby, Cedar Grove (lodging, cafe, small store, campgrounds)
Getting to the Trailhead: Go 85 miles east from Fresno on State Route 180, past Grant Grove Village in Kings Canyon National Park (park headquarters is located here), over a summit, then down into Kings Canyon to Roads End, 6 miles east of Cedar Grove Village.

Baxter Pass Trail

Access to East Side: Independence
Location: 11S 374508E 4077248N; 10,200'
Distance from Endpoints: 170.3 miles from YV; 48.2 miles from WP
Maps: USGS *Mt. Clarence King, Kearsarge Peak;* TH *Kings Canyon High Country*
Permits: INF: Baxter Pass Trailhead
The Hike: 11 miles (allow one to three days); go through Baxter Lakes basin (campsites), then over Baxter Pass (12,320') to descend a long,

unmaintained trail with a few campsites to the end of Oak Creek Road. This is a difficult trail.

Trailhead Amenities: Campground nearby

Getting to the Trailhead: From Independence, head north on Hwy. 395 for 2.5 miles. Turn west onto paved Fish Hatchery Road and go 1.3 miles to a Y-junction. Go right here, passing Oak Creek Campground, to the trailhead, 5.8 miles from the Y-junction. This is a very low-use trail, and finding a ride to Independence is likely to be difficult.

Kearsarge Pass Trail, from North

Access to East Side: Independence

Location: 11S 373529E 4070466N; 10,760'

Distance from Endpoints: 177.3 miles from YV; 41.2 miles from WP (alternative to Charlotte Lake: 177.6 miles from YV; 40.9 miles from WP)

Maps: USGS *Mt. Clarence King, Kearsarge Peak*; TH *Kings Canyon High Country*

Permits: INF: Kearsarge Pass Trailhead

The Hike: 7 miles (allow for one day); head over Kearsarge Pass on a long, dry traverse without campsites, then through an east-side lakes basin, with campsites, to Onion Valley Trailhead. A spur trail, leading to Charlotte Lake, crosses the JMT just to the south and shortly intersects the northern trail over Kearsarge Pass.

Trailhead Amenities: Toilet, water, and campground

Getting to the Trailhead: In Independence, turn west from Hwy. 395 onto Market Street (Onion Valley Road), and follow it for 12.5 steep, winding miles to a large parking area that serves three trailheads. Kearsarge Pass is the middle and most obvious trailhead. For many, this is an ideal location for a resupply, but be sure to schedule in sufficient time to find a ride—especially from Independence back to the trailhead.

Kearsarge Pass Trail, from South

Access to East Side: Independence

Location: 11S 374109E 4069881N; 10,515'

Distance from Endpoints: 178.1 miles from YV; 40.4 miles from WP

Maps: USGS *Mt. Clarence King, Kearsarge Peak*; TH *Kings Canyon High Country*

Permits: INF: Kearsarge Pass Trailhead

The Hike: 7.5 miles (allow for one day); go through the Bullfrog-Kearsarge Basin, past the Kearsarge Lakes (campsites, bear boxes). Then climb steeply to meet the trail from the north junction a little west of Kearsarge Pass. Bullfrog Lake is closed to camping. Continue over

Kearsarge Pass, through an east-side lakes basin to Onion Valley Trailhead.

Trailhead Amenities: Toilet, water, and campground

Getting to the Trailhead: Follow the directions to Kearsarge Pass Trail, from North, on page 233.

Bubbs Creek Trail

Access to West Side: Roads End at Cedar Grove

Location: 11S 374004E 4068999N; 9515'

Distance from Endpoints: 179.4 miles from YV; 39.1 miles from WP

Maps: USGS *Mt. Clarence King, The Sphinx*, TH *Kings Canyon High Country, Mt. Whitney High Country*

Permits: SEKI: Bubbs Creek Trailhead

The Hike: 12 miles (allow one to two days); go west, along Bubbs Creek, to Roads End (Cedar Grove); there are campsites and bear boxes along the way.

Trailhead Amenities: Toilets, National Park Service ranger station and, nearby, Cedar Grove (lodging, cafe, small store, campgrounds)

Getting to the Trailhead: Go 85 miles east from Fresno on State Route 180, past Grant Grove Village in Kings Canyon National Park (park headquarters is located here), over a summit, then down into Kings Canyon to Roads End, 6 miles east of Cedar Grove Village.

Shepherd Pass Trail

Access to East Side: Independence

Location: 11S 376038E 4055756N; 10,890'

Distance from Endpoints: 191.8 miles from YV; 26.7 miles from WP

Maps: USGS *Mt. Williamson*; TH *Mt. Whitney High Country*

Permits: INF: Shepherd Pass Trailhead

The Hike: 12.5 miles (allow one to two days); go over Shepherd Pass (12,050'; snow may linger on the east side) and descend past some campsites to Symmes Creek Trailhead. The trail segment in Sequoia National Park has been reconstructed, while it is in disrepair on the Inyo National Forest side.

Trailhead Amenities: None

Getting to the Trailhead: In Independence, turn from Hwy. 395 west onto Market Street (Onion Valley Road). Go 4.4 miles to Foothill Road, turn left, and go 2.6 miles to a junction. Take the left-hand fork and immediately cross Symmes Creek. In a half mile, take the right fork. At the next two forks, again take the right fork, before continuing 1.6 miles to the trailhead near Symmes Creek. After July 15, this is a relatively low-use trail, and finding a ride to Independence is likely to be difficult.

PCT South, from Crabtree to Cottonwood Lakes

Access to East Side: Lone Pine and the rest of the PCT
Location: 11S 378224E 4046604N; 10,760'
Distance from Endpoints: 199.9 miles from YV; 18.6 miles from WP
Maps: USGS *Mt. Whitney, Johnson Peak, Cirque Lake*; TH *Mt. Whitney High Country*
Permits: INF: Cottonwood Lakes Trailhead
The Hike: 20 miles (allow two to four days); go south along the PCT, up Rock Creek, over New Army Pass (12,315'), and through the Cottonwood Lakes to the Cottonwood Lakes Trailhead. There are campsites and bear boxes along the way.
Trailhead Amenities: Toilets and campground
Getting to the Trailhead: Turn west from Hwy. 395 in Lone Pine onto the Whitney Portal Road. Go 3 miles and turn left onto the Horseshoe Meadow Road. Go 18 miles, past the Cottonwood walk-in campground, to the Cottonwood Lakes parking area. This is an alternative way to begin the JMT if you cannot get a permit to begin the hike out of Whitney Portal.

Nearby Towns

The following towns are accessible from the JMT lateral trails. They are listed from north to south.

Yosemite Valley: Lodging, restaurants, campgrounds, groceries, mountaineering and sporting goods store, and post office.
Tuolumne Meadows (Yosemite National Park): Lodging, small cafe, campground, groceries, small mountaineering and sporting goods store, and post office.
Lee Vining: Small town with lodging, restaurants, groceries, and post office.
June Lake: Small town with lodging, restaurants, campgrounds, groceries, and post office.
Mammoth Lakes: Town with ample lodging, restaurants, campgrounds, groceries, mountaineering and sporting goods stores, and post office. Ranks with Bishop as your best choice if you must go out to a town to resupply.
Bishop: Town with ample lodging, restaurants, campgrounds, groceries, mountaineering and sporting goods stores, and post office. Ranks with Mammoth Lakes as your best choice if you must go out to a town to resupply.
Big Pine: Small town with lodging, restaurants, a campground, some groceries, and post office.

Independence: Small town with lodging, restaurants, a campground, some groceries, and post office.

Lone Pine: Small town with lodging, restaurants, some groceries, small mountaineering and sporting goods stores, and post office.

Resupply Locations

The following resorts and post offices are good places to send your packages or stock up on some supplies.

Reds Meadow Resort

Accessed from Reds Meadow Resort junction. The resort offers lodging, camping, a cafe, and a store (they sell stove fuel). They accept both hand-delivered and mailed resupply packages in boxes.

Contact Information:

Red's Meadow
PO Box 395
Mammoth Lakes, CA 93546
760-934-2345 or 800-292-7758
www.redsmeadow.com
rmps395@aol.com

Food Box Costs: $1 per day for hand-delivered packages; $25 plus $1 per day after the first five days for mailed packages. See www.redsmeadow.com/pdf/PackagePickUp.pdf for additional regulations and services.

Vermilion Valley Resort

Accessed from Lake Edison, Bear Ridge, and Bear Creek trails. The shortest distance from the JMT, via Lake Edison Trail and Lake Edison Ferry (twice daily, $18 round trip) is 2.5 miles round trip. The resort offers lodging, camping, a cafe, and a store (they sell stove fuel). They accept mailed resupply packages, preferably by USPS. As a bonus, thru-hikers get their first beer free.

Contact Information for USPS:

Vermilion Valley Resort
PO Box 258
Lakeshore, CA 93634

Contact Information for United Parcel Service:

Vermilion Valley Resort
c/o Rancheria Garage
62311 Huntington Lake Road

Lakeshore, CA 93634
559-259-4000 (seasonal, at the resort)
www.edisonlake.com
info@edisonlake.com

Food Box Costs: $15 per 25-pound package. See www.edisonlake.
com/resupply.htm for additional regulations and services.

Muir Trail Ranch

Accessed from Florence Lake Trail. The shortest distance from the
JMT is a half mile round trip, once you reach the junction between the
two JMT cutoffs. The resort stores mailed food packages and has an
excellent collection of "leftover food" buckets for hikers to rummage
through or deposit into. Their small store carries stove fuel, batter-
ies, and postcards. Their lodging and food are reserved for their own
guests. However, there are campsites nearby and a free hot-spring pool
across the river (the ford may be very dangerous in early season).

Contact Information for Summer:

Muir Trail Ranch
PO Box 176
Lakeshore, CA 93634

Contact Information for Off-Season:

PO Box 269
Ahwahnee, CA 93601
209-966-3195 (office in Ahwahnee; no phone at resort)
www.muirtrailranch.com
resupply@muirtrailranch.com

Food Box Costs: $50 per white plastic bucket. See www.muirtrail-
ranch.com/resupply.html for additional regulations and services.

Post Offices

There are post offices in all the east-side towns accessible from the
JMT. The business hours, street address, and phone numbers for these
post offices can be found at www.usps.com. The only post office near
a trailhead on the west side of the range is at the General Store at the
Mono Hot Springs Resort, accessed from the Lake Edison Trail, Bear
Ridge Trail, and Bear Creek Trail. Additional information on the Mono
Hot Springs Post Office is available by calling 209-325-1710, or by visit-
ing www.monohotsprings.com/post.html.

Post offices are legally required to hold your packages for only 10 days, so be sure to contact them ahead of time if your package will be there for a longer period of time. Be sure to specify a "hold until" date on the box.

When mailing your package to any of these places, address it to:

[Yourself]
c/o General Delivery
[post office], CA [zip]
HOLD UNTIL [date]

Post offices in towns along the JMT follow, in north-to-south order:

Yosemite Valley Post Office
Yosemite National Park, CA 95389-9998

Tuolumne Meadows Post Office
Yosemite National Park, CA 95389-9906

Lee Vining Post Office
Lee Vining, CA 93541-9997

June Lake Post Office
June Lake, CA 93529-9997

Mammoth Lakes Post Office
Mammoth Lakes, CA 93546-9997

Bishop Post Office
Bishop, CA 93514-9998

Big Pine Post Office
Big Pine, CA 93513-9997

Independence Post Office
Independence, CA 93526-9997

Lone Pine Post Office
Lone Pine, CA 93545-9997

Mono Hot Springs
Mono Hot Springs, CA 93642

Resupply Using Packstock

An alternative resupply option is to have your food carried in by one of the pack stations operating in the eastern Sierra Nevada. Known as a "dunnage drop" by the packers, this would simplify your resupply logistics along the southern half of the JMT. Food drops can easily be arranged for Le Conte Canyon or at the Kearsarge Pass junction. Per-day costs are approximately $95 per mule (each mule can carry up to 150 pounds of food) and $210 per packer.

Rainbow Pack Outfitters provides service over Bishop Pass and down to Le Conte Canyon. This is a two-day round trip for the packer. You can halve your costs by meeting the packer atop Bishop Pass:

PO Box 1791
Bishop, CA 93515
760-873-8877 (pack station)
760-872-8803 (office)
760-873-7523 (fax)
www.rainbowoutfitters.com

Sequoia Kings Pack Trains provides service over Kearsarge Pass and down to the John Muir Trail at the Charlotte Lake junction:

PO Box 209
Independence, CA 93526
800-962-0775
760-387-2797
760-387-2627 (fax)

Other pack stations based in the eastern Sierra are listed at: www. fs.fed.us/r5/inyo/recreation/packstations.shtml.

APPENDIX C.

Campsites

The following chart provides a selection of campsites along the JMT. It is not comprehensive, but it includes most campsites that are visible from the trail. Lacking fire rings, campsites above treeline tend to be smaller and more hidden; a few are included here, but more can be found with a little searching. A disclaimer: UTM coordinates may be off by as much as 100 feet (30 meters), especially in deep canyons or forested areas.

Camp ID	N–S	S–N	Elevation	UTM Coordinates (NAD27)	Description
CAMP 1.01	4.4	13.9	6130	11S 278409E 4179015N	Large camping area in eastern Little Yosemite Valley; bear boxes; toilet
CAMP 1.02	6.5	11.8	7190	11S 279498E 4180201N	At Clouds Rest junction; camping both adjacent to creek and on granite knob to northwest of trail junction
CAMP 1.03	6.6	11.7	7215	11S 279571E 4180130N	Large camping area by Sunrise Creek; opening in white fir forest
CAMP 1.04	6.7	11.6	7240	11S 279662E 4180209N	Open knob to west of trail under open Jeffrey pine cover; large area with excellent views to Half Dome
CAMP 1.05	6.9	11.4	7375	11S 279943E 4180163N	Large opening south of trail in Jeffrey pine/white fir forest; alongside granite outcrops
CAMP 1.06	7.0	11.3	7410	11S 280211E 4180245N	Large opening south of trail in Jeffrey pine/white fir forest
CAMP 1.07	7.3	11.0	7520	11S 280420E 4180418N	Just west of creek crossing, head up use trail to the north; sites with excellent vistas to the west and more sheltered sites in Jeffrey pine/white fir forest to the east; excellent sites
CAMP 1.08	7.7	10.6	7720	11S 281011E 4180674N	Opening in white fir forest alongside Sunrise Creek

Camp ID	N–S	S–N	Elevation	UTM Coordinates (NAD27)	Description
CAMP 1.09	8.0	10.3	7800	11S 281363E 4180922N	A little knob with room for several tents
CAMP 1.10	8.1	10.2	7825	11S 281350E 4181052N	Large opening west of creek in white fir forest; nice site
CAMP 1.11	10.2	8.1	8520	11S 284046E 4182357N	Along a side creek that may be dry in late season; large opening in white fir forest
CAMP 1.12	10.3	8.0	8540	11S 284017E 4182458N	Large opening in dense forest alongside Sunrise Creek; other options farther upstream
CAMP 1.13	12.0	6.3	9590	11S 285081E 4184074N	Large flat area to the south of the trail, beneath open lodgepole cover at the edge of a large meadow
CAMP 1.14	12.0	6.3	9585	11S 285199E 4184108N	Sandy flat area to the north of the trail, at the edge of slabs beneath scattered lodgepole pines
CAMP 1.15	12.1	6.2	9585	11S 285348E 4184149N	Sandy flat area to the south of the trail, beneath open lodgepole cover at the edge of a large meadow
CAMP 1.16	12.8	5.5	9330	11S 285635E 4184995N	To the east of creek beneath hemlocks and a few lodgepole pines; excellent views
CAMP 1.17	13.1	5.2	9310	11S 285790E 4185522N	Sunrise High Sierra Camp camping area; head up trail toward sunrise lakes to find many camping options on both sides of the trail; toilet
CAMP 1.18	14.1	4.2	9320	11S 286135E 4186602N	Camping area with fire ring just north of the Echo Creek Junction, on a small knob to the west of the trail
CAMP 1.19	17.0	1.3	9595	11S 287714E 4190414N	Small sites to the eastern edge of the meadow on slabs beneath scattered lodgepole pines
CAMP 1.20	17.2	1.1	9600	11S 287744E 4190680N	Sandy flats among slabs at the northern edge of the upper Cathedral Lake; excellent views
CAMP 1.21	17.3	1.0	9600	11S 287735E 4190733N	Opening in lodgepole forest just north of the upper Cathedral Lake and adjacent meadow
CAMP 1.22	17.8	0.5	9425	11S 287610E 4191528N	Many picturesque sites available at the lower Cathedral Lakes, 0.5 mile off the trail

Camp ID	N–S	S–N	Elevation	UTM Coordinates (NAD27)	Description
CAMP 2.01	4.6	13.5	8585	11S 293079E 4194157N	Tuolumne Meadows backpacker's campground
CAMP 2.02	10.0	8.1	8840	11S 298953E 4190552N	Avalanche zone that marks beginning of legal camping in Lyell Canyon
CAMP 2.03	11.2	6.9	8900	11S 299472E 4188756N	Many sites in openings in lodgepole forest to the northwest of the Evelyn Lake Trail junction
CAMP 2.04	13.7	4.4	8990	11S 300902E 4185497N	Large area in opening in lodgepole forest to the west of trail; additional smaller sites nearby
CAMP 2.05	14.3	3.9	9030	11S 300914E 4184682N	At beginning of climb out of Lyell Canyon, opening in lodgepole forest
CAMP 2.06	15.1	3.0	9700	11S 300788E 4183634N	Flat area among hemlocks and lodgepole pines to the west of the bridge crossing
CAMP 2.07	15.2	2.9	9680	11S 300845E 4183438N	Flat area among hemlocks and lodgepole pines to the east of the bridge crossing
CAMP 2.08	16.3	1.8	10,190	11S 301348E 4182280N	Several small sites under stunted whitebark pines to the northeast of the lake
CAMP 2.09	16.8	1.3	10,535	11S 301125E 4181600N	Few small exposed sites in sandy patches among slabs
CAMP 3.01	1.5	3.4	10,370	11S 303600E 4181503N	Search for small, sandy sites on knobs above the otherwise meadow-covered ground; beautiful views
CAMP 3.02	2.7	2.2	10,040	11S 304471E 4180124N	Large area just south of Marie Lakes junction
CAMP 3.03	3.4	1.5	9640	11S 305090E 4179708N	Flat area on knob to west of trail, north of the Rush Creek forks
CAMP 4.01	0.3	22.2	10,230	11S 306896E 4178362N	Small sites to the edge of the lakes on Island Pass
CAMP 4.02	1.8	20.7	9830	11S 308736E 4177715N	Head along the use trail west from the Thousand Island Lake junction; sites to the north of the trail in sandy patches among granite slabs; camping prohibited within 0.25 mile of outlet
CAMP 4.03	2.0	20.5	9830	11S 308969E 4177501N	Several sites on the knob to the southwest of the Thousand Island Lake outlet; camping prohibited within 0.25 mile of outlet

Camp ID	N–S	S–N	Elevation	UTM Coordinates (NAD27)	Description
CAMP 4.04	2.8	19.7	9900	11S 309754E 4176911N	Small site just southeast of Ruby Lake outlet; under open hemlock cover
CAMP 4.05	3.7	18.8	9700	11S 310179E 4176014N	Large site along the shores of Garnet Lake; scattered tree cover and excellent views; additional sites farther west along the northern shore of Garnet Lake
CAMP 4.06	4.2	18.3	9700	11S 310424E 4175817N	Small sites along the southern shore of Garnet Lake; small flat sections on an otherwise steep slope; excellent views
CAMP 4.07	4.7	17.8	10,100	11S 310509E 4175326N	A few small, open sites to the southwest of the tarn on the pass south of Garnet Lake
CAMP 4.08	5.9	16.6	9170	11S 310679E 4173859N	Large, open sites in lodgepole/ western white pine forest to the edge of the creek
CAMP 4.09	6.2	16.3	9100	11S 310870E 4173637N	Large, open sites in lodgepole/ western white pine forest to the edge of the creek; surrounded by small granite outcrops
CAMP 4.10	8.8	13.7	9350	11S 313018E 4173111N	Medium-sized sites in wet hemlock forest to the south of the Rosalie Lake outlet
CAMP 4.11	9.5	13.0	9570	11S 313256E 4172369N	Medium-sized sites in forest opening along the southwestern edge of Gladys Lake
CAMP 4.12	10.3	12.2	9400	11S 313736E 4171490N	Large, sandy sites to the west of the trail; water nearby from the Trinity Lakes
CAMP 4.13	14.2	8.3	8100	11S 315197E 4167922N	Sites in open lodgepole forest to the north of the Minaret Creek crossing; beautiful cobbled creek
CAMP 4.14	15.0	7.5	7680	11S 315747E 4166939N	Head east from the northern Devils Postpile junction to the Devils Postpile campground
CAMP 4.15	17.4	5.1	7720	11S 316900E 4164357N	Head north from the Reds Meadow junction to the Reds Meadow campground
CAMP 4.16	20.5	2.0	8640	11S 318381E 4162299N	A few small sites on knobs to the northeast of the Crater Creek crossing
CAMP 4.17	20.5	2.0	8635	11S 318312E 4162198N	Several small sites in forest openings to the southwest of the Crater Creek crossing

Camp ID	N–S	S–N	Elevation	UTM Coordinates (NAD27)	Description
CAMP 4.18	21.4	1.1	8915	11S 319327E 4161594N	Head east from the Mammoth Pass junction in Upper Crater Meadows; sites along the northeastern and eastern meadow edge
CAMP 5.01	0.9	16.4	9100	11S 320408E 4159174N	Large site just to the north of the Deer Creek crossing in open lodgepole forest; other sites nearby
CAMP 5.02	6.3	11.0	9970	11S 325841E 4156281N	Small sites in stand of trees just upslope of trail; open view to the Silver Divide
CAMP 5.03	6.3	11.0	9990	11S 325876E 4156259N	Small sites among slabs to the edge of creek draining Duck Creek; parallel creek downstream to find several choices
CAMP 5.04	8.6	8.7	9970	11S 327744E 4155131N	Sites along the west shore of Purple Lake; take spur trail north of crossing
CAMP 5.05	10.6	6.7	10,350	11S 329103E 4153669N	Sites nestled among stunted whitebark pines to the northwest of Virginia Lake
CAMP 5.06	12.7	4.6	9550	11S 330075E 4152142N	Large stock site just north of Tully Hole junction beneath open lodgepole pines
CAMP 5.07	13.0	4.3	9500	11S 329661E 4151738N	Medium-sized site in open lodgepole forest along a stretch of Fish Creek with big pools and slabs
CAMP 5.08	13.7	3.6	9200	11S 329256E 4151042N	Large site in hemlock and fir forest, a bit south of Fish Creek bridge
CAMP 5.09	13.7	3.6	9200	11S 329204E 4150952N	Site on open knob just north of Fish Creek junction
CAMP 5.10	14.2	3.1	9500	11S 329067E 4150517N	Small sites among heath vegetation and hemlocks, on flatter section of climb
CAMP 5.11	14.8	2.5	9760	11S 328994E 4149815N	Sites in trees to edge of small marsh; just south of bridge crossing
CAMP 5.12	15.7	1.6	10,300	11S 329958E 4149436N	Small, sandy sites among slabs, mostly on the north side of Squaw Lake outlet; open views and evening sun
CAMP 5.13	16.4	0.9	10,560	11S 329612E 4148847N	Sites among slabs to the edge of meadows surrounding tarns near Chief Lake; open with just a few whitebark pines

Camp ID	N–S	S–N	Elevation	UTM Coordinates (NAD27)	Description
CAMP 5.14	16.8	0.5	10,780	11S 329960E 4148900N	Large, exposed, sandy areas for the next 0.2 mile, many with nearby water until late season, beautiful views of the basin
CAMP 6.01	0.8	19.5	10,420	11S 330215E 4147233N	Small, scattered sites along Silver Lake among lodgepole pines
CAMP 6.02	2.3	18	9840	11S 330007E 4145514N	Open, forested site along creek with lodgepole pines and a few hemlock
CAMP 6.03	3.7	16.6	8980	11S 331341E 4145024N	Small site beneath forest cover near the Mott Lake junction
CAMP 6.04	5.2	15.1	8310	11S 330981E 4143088N	Open, forested site beneath Jeffrey pines
CAMP 6.05	6.5	13.8	7900	11S 329754E 4142197N	Large, open area beneath Jeffrey pines at junction with Lake Thomas Edison Trail
CAMP 6.06	11.7	8.6	9520	11S 331399E 4138386N	Small site with beautiful views and junipers on descent to Bear Creek
CAMP 6.07	11.9	8.4	9480	11S 331557E 4138305N	Larger site shaded by large Jeffrey pines
CAMP 6.08	13.8	6.5	9080	11S 333367E 4136566N	Large site in open lodgepole forest along Bear Creek
CAMP 6.09	14.3	6	9160	11S 333635E 4135829N	Large site in open lodgepole forest along Bear Creek
CAMP 6.10	14.7	5.6	9240	11S 333740E 4135259N	Large site in open lodgepole forest along Bear Creek
CAMP 6.11	15.1	5.2	9290	11S 333764E 4134777N	Site in open lodgepole forest along Bear Creek
CAMP 6.12	15.2	5.1	9320	11S 333943E 4134624N	Site in open lodgepole forest along the Hilgard Branch
CAMP 6.13	16.1	4.2	9550	11S 334527E 4133430N	Site in wetter forest along Bear Creek, 200 feet west of trail
CAMP 6.14	16.4	3.9	9580	11S 334696E 4133064N	Site in open lodgepole forest near Bear Creek crossing
CAMP 6.15	17.5	2.8	10,010	11S 334421E 4131834N	Site in opening south of stream crossing, possible muddy
CAMP 6.16	17.7	2.6	10,030	11S 334322E 4131553N	Sites on slabs to the side of Rosemarie Meadow
CAMP 6.17	19.5	0.8	10,570	11S 334213E 4129661N	Small, sandy sites among slabs and whitebark pines along Marie Lake

Camp ID	N–S	S–N	Elevation	UTM Coordinates (NAD27)	Description
CAMP 7.01	0.7	25.8	10,550	11S 333912E 4127505N	Small, exposed sites on slabs near Heart Lake; must leave trail to find; beautiful views
CAMP 7.02	1.5	25.0	10,200	11S 333799E 4126475N	Many large sites beneath lodgepole pines between the Sallie Keyes Lakes
CAMP 7.03	1.7	24.8	10,200	11S 333710E 4126334N	Large site beneath lodgepole pines near the Sallie Keyes outlet
CAMP 7.04	2.5	24.0	10,000	11S 333875E 4125232N	Site in open lodgepole forest
CAMP 7.05	2.8	23.7	10,100	11S 334037E 4125004N	Site on knob with a beautiful view; water is along the trail just to the south
CAMP 7.06	3.6	22.9	9750	11S 334684E 4124402N	Site in lodgepole forest along Senger Creek; respect posted "no camping" areas
CAMP 7.07	7.4	19.1	7800	11S 334425E 4121699N	Small site on a shelf along Piute Creek, on south cutoff to Muir Trail Ranch
CAMP 7.08	7.4	19.1	7780	11S 334532E 4121551N	Large site along Piute Creek, on south cutoff to Muir Trail Ranch
CAMP 7.09	9.2	17.3	8070	11S 337454E 4121242N	Large site beneath open Jeffrey Pines on the south side of the bridge at the Piute Pass junction
CAMP 7.10	9.7	16.8	8110	11S 338004E 4120820N	Small site along a dry, rocky section of Piute Creek
CAMP 7.11	10.6	15.9	8200	11S 338794E 4119983N	Large site amongst aspen, lodgepoles, and white fir; similar site just upstream
CAMP 7.12	10.7	15.8	8210	11S 338899E 4119894N	Small, open site beneath a magnificent juniper
CAMP 7.13	10.7	15.8	8230	11S 339039E 4119835N	Small, open site on a shelf just north of Aspen Creek crossing
CAMP 7.14	11.8	14.7	8380	11S 340245E 4118705N	Large area beneath lodgepole pines along Piute Creek; follow spur trail just south of bridge
CAMP 7.15	12.0	14.5	8420	11S 340458E 4118467N	Various camping options along a flat section in wetter lodgepole forest
CAMP 7.16	12.8	13.7	8460	11S 340790E 4117649N	Sandy, open site just to south of bridge crossing
CAMP 7.17	12.9	13.6	8460	11S 340778E 4117859N	Site in wet lodgepole forest at base of switchbacks
CAMP 7.18	14.4	12.1	9225	11S 342097E 4117967N	Site in lodgepole forest along section with lots of small creeks

Camp ID	N–S	S–N	Elevation	UTM Coordinates (NAD27)	Description
CAMP 7.19	14.8	11.7	9230	11S 342680E 4117857N	Site in lodgepole forest at the edge of Evolution Meadow
CAMP 7.20	16.0	10.5	9540	11S 344612E 4117060N	Site in open lodgepole forest
CAMP 7.21	16.4	10.1	9630	11S 345071E 4116992N	Several medium-sized sites at the western end of McClure Meadow; beautiful views to Mt. Darwin and the Hermit
CAMP 7.22	16.7	9.8	9640	11S 345489E 4116942N	Several small- to large-sized sites toward the eastern end of McClure Meadow; beautiful views to Mt. Darwin and the Hermit
CAMP 7.23	17.4	9.1	9730	11S 346408E 4116509N	Site in open lodgepole forest
CAMP 7.24	18.7	7.8	9960	11S 347942E 4115371N	Site on open slabs just south of the Darwin Bench drainage
CAMP 7.25	22.5	4.0	11,140	11S 349752E 4112189N	Open sites near the inlet to Sapphire Lake; these sites are 200 feet below the trail; picturesque
CAMP 8.01	3.1	18.6	10,840	11S 354202E 4109547N	Several small sites among whitebark pines at outlet to Lake 10,800+ feet; excellent views
CAMP 8.02	3.5	18.2	10,640	11S 354369E 4109065N	Large site beneath lodgepole pines with views to the Black Giant
CAMP 8.03	3.7	18.0	10,480	11S 354401E 4108820N	Large site beneath lodgepole pines with views to the Black Giant
CAMP 8.04	4.0	17.7	10,320	11S 354585E 4108611N	Starr Camp; lots of good sites among young lodgepole pines to the south of the trail; beautiful views of Languille Peak, the Black Giant, and Le Conte Canyon
CAMP 8.05	5.2	16.5	9470	11S 356035E 4108398N	Medium-sized site beside creek just south of the switchbacks
CAMP 8.06	5.5	16.2	9380	11S 356450E 4108404N	Large, well-used site in opening in lodgepole forest
CAMP 8.07	5.8	15.9	9310	11S 356935E 4108493N	Medium-sized, well-used site in opening in lodgepole forest
CAMP 8.08	6.1	15.6	9240	11S 357367E 4108395N	Several small sites in openings in lodgepole forest just south of creek crossing
CAMP 8.09	6.3	15.4	9230	11S 357582E 4108192N	Big Pete Meadow; lateral trail to large site by creek under lodgepole cover
CAMP 8.10	6.8	14.9	8990	11S 357840E 4107634N	Handful of small sites on granite knob with junipers; view to Languille Peak

Camp ID	N–S	S–N	Elevation	UTM Coordinates (NAD27)	Description
CAMP 8.11	7.2	14.5	8870	11S 358043E 4107209N	Little Pete Meadow; medium-sized site on edge of meadow with meandering river; view to Languille Peak
CAMP 8.12	8.0	13.7	8700	11S 358442E 4106162N	Sites on both sides of the trail, to the east a small site on slabs, to the west a larger site beneath lodgepoles
CAMP 8.13	8.0	13.7	8700	11S 358432E 4106123N	Medium-sized site beneath lodgepoles
CAMP 8.14	8.3	13.4	8650	11S 358291E 4105747N	Site in opening in lodgepole forest just to the edge of avalanche path
CAMP 8.15	8.4	13.3	8640	11S 358326E 4105634N	Site in opening in lodgepole forest just to the edge of avalanche path
CAMP 8.16	10.2	11.5	8260	11S 358786E 4102849N	Large site at the edge of Grouse Meadow in opening beneath lodgepole; open views of Le Conte Canyon; many options nearby
CAMP 8.17	10.3	11.4	8260	11S 358914E 4102788N	Medium-sized site at the edge of Grouse Meadow in opening beneath lodgepole; open views of Le Conte Canyon; many options nearby
CAMP 8.18	11.2	10.5	8060	11S 359606E 4101694N	Several large sites beneath Jeffrey pines at the Middle Fork Trail junction
CAMP 8.19	12.4	9.3	8410	11S 361072E 4101674N	Large site beside slow-flowing river; meadows and open Jeffrey pine forest
CAMP 8.20	12.6	9.1	8420	11S 361315E 4101663N	Small site beneath open Jeffrey pines
CAMP 8.21	13.7	8.0	8615	11S 362899E 4101649N	Medium-sized site in open, sandy area
CAMP 8.22	14.0	7.7	8680	11S 363370E 4101720N	Large site to the edge of burn area, surrounded by meadows and open Jeffrey pines
CAMP 8.23	14.3	7.4	8730	11S 363706E 4101862N	Small site to the edge of burn area, surrounded by meadows and open Jeffrey pines
CAMP 8.24	14.7	7.0	8900	11S 364381E 4101948N	Deer Meadow; large site beneath lodgepole forest at Deer Creek crossing
CAMP 8.25	15.2	6.5	8920	11S 365025E 4101807N	Medium-sized site beneath lodgepole forest toward base of the Golden Staircase

Camp ID	N–S	S–N	Elevation	UTM Coordinates (NAD27)	Description
CAMP 8.26	15.5	6.2	8980	11S 365390E 4101802N	Medium-sized site beneath lodgepole forest toward base of the Golden Staircase
CAMP 8.27	18.2	3.5	10,630	11S 367770E 4102381N	Several medium-sized sandy sites to edge of slabs at the lower Palisade Lake outlet; beautiful views to the west and to the middle Palisades
CAMP 8.28	19.1	2.6	10,860	11S 368854E 4101944N	Small, sandy tent sites beneath stunted whitebark pines and overlooking the upper Palisade Lake; excellent views; by late season, water could be a five-minute walk upstream
CAMP 8.29	19.4	2.3	10,860	11S 369102E 4101754N	Several medium-sized, sandy sites beneath stunted whitebark pines and overlooking the upper Palisade Lake; excellent views; water a short distance south on trail
CAMP 8.30	19.5	2.2	10,880	11S 369255E 4101493N	Small, sandy tent sites beneath stunted whitebark pines and overlooking the upper Palisade Lake; excellent views
CAMP 9.01	1.3	8.5	11,500	11S 370474E 4098256N	Ample sites among small tarns in Upper Basin
CAMP 9.02	3.9	5.9	10,560	11S 371175E 4094329N	One of many sites to the east of the trail, in sandy patches toward stream; open lodgepole forest
CAMP 9.03	4.7	5.1	10,280	11S 371635E 4093173N	One of many sites to the east of the trail, in sandy patches toward stream; open lodgepole forest
CAMP 9.04	4.9	4.9	10,195	11S 371678E 4092862N	Site beneath lodgepole forest and near stream; at unmarked junction with old lateral trail to Taboose Pass
CAMP 9.05	5.2	4.6	10,040	11S 371517E 4092357N	Site in lodgepole forest to the east of the trail, near stream; restoration area to the west
CAMP 9.06	5.3	4.5	10,070	11S 371539E 4092284N	Large site in lodgepole forest on south side of stream crossing
CAMP 9.07	7.0	2.8	10,850	11S 372169E 4091050N	A few small sites near the trail among scattered trees; views north
CAMP 9.08	7.3	2.5	11,000	11S 372287E 4090591N	A few medium-sized sites near the trail among scattered trees; views north
CAMP 9.09	8.0	1.8	11,130	11S 372593E 4089824N	Small sites among whitebark pines at and below Lake Marjorie outlet

Camp ID	N–S	S–N	Elevation	UTM Coordinates (NAD27)	Description
CAMP 9.10	8.5	1.3	11,250	11S 373097E 4089328N	Small, exposed site; beautiful views
CAMP 10.01	1.5	14.4	11,350	11S 375438E 4087442N	Small, sandy sites among whitebark pines; additional sites next to tarns to the northeast of the trail
CAMP 10.02	2.7	13.2	10,910	11S 375732E 4086052N	Large site on knob to the east of trail, in mixed lodgepole and whitebark pine forest; additional smaller sites nearby
CAMP 10.03	3.7	12.2	10,350	11S 375312E 4084783N	Small site at Sawmill Trail junction, just east of creek crossing; under lodgepole cover with wet streamside vegetation
CAMP 10.04	4.4	11.5	9840	11S 374422E 4084480N	Large site in lodgepole forest
CAMP 10.05	5.6	10.3	9235	11S 373434E 4083321N	One larger site with a fire ring and a few other sites with space for a single tent on an open knob with scattered Jeffrey pines
CAMP 10.06	7.3	8.6	8530	11S 371951E 4081607N	Large site just south of Woods Creek Crossing with room for 20 parties; additional sites on the knob to the southwest of the trail; bear boxes
CAMP 10.07	9.6	6.3	9500	11S 374105E 4079237N	Small sites visible from trail and large ones if you head north; at the edge of a moist meadow
CAMP 10.08	11.0	4.9	10,200	11S 374543E 4077245N	Several sites to the north of Dollar Lake; beautiful reflections of Fin Dome in the lake
CAMP 10.09	11.0	4.9	10,220	11S 374454E 4077222N	Sites to the west of trail, behind boulders; follow use trail just south of Baxter Pass junction
CAMP 10.10	11.6	4.3	10,300	11S 374349E 4076467N	Many sites along Arrowhead Lake; some in open lodgepole forest and others on open sandier knobs; excellent views to Fin Dome; bear box
CAMP 10.11	12.6	3.4	10,550	11S 374712E 4075148N	Large sites under sparse lodgepole cover; excellent Rae Lakes views
CAMP 10.12	12.6	3.3	10,560	11S 374736E 4075047N	Large sites under sparse lodgepole cover; excellent Rae Lakes views; bear box
CAMP 10.13	13.1	2.8	10,590	11S 375190E 4074578N	Small site on open, sandy slabs, high above the water; excellent views

Camp ID	N–S	S–N	Elevation	UTM Coordinates (NAD27)	Description
CAMP 10.14	13.4	2.5	10,600	11S 375346E 4074143N	Many sites in open, sandy areas between scattered lodgepole pines; follow marked use trail west toward the lake; bear box
CAMP 10.15	14.0	1.9	10,580	11S 374962E 4073715N	Open, sandy sites near 60 Lakes junction; look on slope directly west of junction and slightly north along the 60 Lakes Basin Trail; good views to the Painted Lady and the Rae Lakes
CAMP 10.16	14.8	1.1	11,090	11S 374545E 4073104N	Small site among whitebark pines on knob to east of trail
CAMP 10.17	15.2	0.7	11,380	11S 374325E 4072693N	Exposed, alpine sites in sandy patches between slabs by tarns to west of trail; sites best seen when you are slightly above them
CAMP 11.01	0.4	11.4	11,580	11S 373961E 4071910N	Small, sandy, exposed sites among stunted whitebark pines; by lake
CAMP 11.02	2.3	9.5	10,740	11S 372780E 4070954N	Large area in lodgepole forest at the north end of Charlotte Lake; bear box; approximately 1 mile off JMT
CAMP 11.03	2.8	9.0	10,510	11S 374109E 4069881N	Small sites among streamside vegetation and foxtails just north of Bullfrog Lake junction
CAMP 11.04	3.0	8.8	10,365	11S 374160E 4069652N	Small site next to creek crossing; lodgepole forest and wet streamside heath vegetation
CAMP 11.05	3.4	8.4	10,070	11S 374397E 4069456N	Medium-sized site beneath lodgepole forest west of creek crossing
CAMP 11.06	4.1	7.7	9510	11S 374020E 4068998N	Large sites in lodgepole forest at Vidette Creek junction
CAMP 11.07	4.3	7.5	9500	11S 374347E 4068984N	Large site in dry lodgepole forest just north of Vidette Meadow
CAMP 11.08	4.4	7.4	9550	11S 374432E 4068927N	Large site that is across Bubbs Creek from the JMT; only accessible by wading stream
CAMP 11.09	4.5	7.3	9550	11S 374522E 4068883N	Several large sites in opening in dry lodgepole forest at edge of Vidette Meadow; views to East Vidette; bear box
CAMP 11.10	4.6	7.2	9560	11S 374684E 4068800N	Large site in dry lodgepole forest at edge of Vidette Meadow; views to East Vidette

Camp ID	N–S	S–N	Elevation	UTM Coordinates (NAD27)	Description
CAMP 11.11	5.3	6.5	9945	11S 375571E 4068228N	Several large sites in opening in dry lodgepole forest; bear boxes
CAMP 11.12	5.5	6.3	9970	11S 375824E 4068146N	Large site in dry lodgepole forest
CAMP 11.13	6.8	5.0	10,380	11S 376948E 4066477N	Small site along stream
CAMP 11.14	7.1	4.7	10,450	11S 377154E 4066134N	Small, sandy sites among slabs a short walk from the bear box
CAMP 11.15	7.2	4.6	10,500	11S 377250E 4066052N	Large, open sites; bear box
CAMP 11.16	7.4	4.4	10,545	11S 377493E 4065693N	Large site in forest near Center Basin Creek crossing
CAMP 11.17	8.3	3.5	10,920	11S 377619E 4064554N	Medium-sized site on sandy knob, among whitebark pines; excellent views
CAMP 11.18	8.3	3.5	10,935	11S 377543E 4064461N	Medium-sized site on sandy knob, among whitebark pines; excellent views
CAMP 11.19	8.8	3.0	11,230	11S 377547E 4063749N	Medium-sized site beneath last stand of stunted whitebark pines; excellent views
CAMP 11.20	8.9	2.9	11,235	11S 377589E 4063735N	Small, exposed, sandy site on edge of alpine meadow; excellent views
CAMP 11.21	9.7	2.1	11,770	11S 378117E 4063444N	Open, sandy site among slabs to the side of a small alpine meadows
CAMP 11.22	10.5	1.3	12,250	11S 377826E 4062513N	Small tent and bivy sites in sandy patches between talus; beautiful views of Junction Peak
CAMP 12.01	0.6	22.6	12,500	11S 377311E 4061261N	Small, exposed sandy sites with views to the Kaweahs
CAMP 12.02	4.5	18.7	10,965	11S 376038E 4055999N	Tyndall Creek crossing; large site under open lodgepole pines along Tyndall Creek; bear box
CAMP 12.03	4.8	18.4	10,880	11S 375984E 4055652N	Large site under open lodgepole pines at Tyndall Creek Trail junction
CAMP 12.04	5.4	17.8	11,025	11S 376211E 4055106N	Tyndall Frog Ponds; large site under open lodgepole pines; bear box
CAMP 12.05	6.7	16.5	11,400	11S 376509E 4053193N	Large, exposed, sandy sites to the north of the pond on Bighorn Plateau; outstanding views
CAMP 12.06	8.3	14.9	10,790	11S 377302E 4051319N	Various sites along Wrights Creek under open lodgepole cover; north of crossing

Camp ID	N–S	S–N	Elevation	UTM Coordinates (NAD27)	Description
CAMP 12.07	8.6	14.6	10,690	11S 377081E 4050931N	Various sites at Wrights Creek crossing, under open lodgepole pines; both sides of crossing
CAMP 12.08	9.3	13.9	10,400	11S 377434E 4050540N	Large site on the north side of the Wallace Creek crossing, adjacent to open meadow
CAMP 12.09	9.3	13.9	10,400	11S 377465E 4050482N	Large site on the south side of the Wallace Creek crossing, under open lodgepole pines; bear box
CAMP 12.10	9.7	13.5	10,650	11S 377508E 4050199N	Single site adjacent to small bubbling creek, under open foxtail and lodgepole pines
CAMP 12.11	10.4	12.8	10,880	11S 377395E 4049396N	Many sites on many nearby sandy flats beneath open foxtail pine cover; beautiful views; only practical if water is available in seasonal streams
CAMP 12.12	11.1	12.1	10,775	11S 377170E 4048376N	Large sites along the northwest side of Sandy Meadow; you must leave the trail to find these
CAMP 12.13	11.3	11.9	10,700	11S 377404E 4048184N	Site at edge of Sandy Meadow in mixed foxtail and lodgepole forest
CAMP 12.14	13.5	9.7	10,690	11S 379147E 4047180N	Large site under lodgepole pine forest
CAMP 12.15	13.6	9.6	10,700	11S 379242E 4047254N	Many large sites around the edge of Crabtree Meadow; take the junction toward the ranger station to the large meadow 0.2 mile to the south; bear box; pit toilet
CAMP 12.16	14.0	9.2	10,735	11S 379729E 4047547N	Large site under lodgepole pine forest
CAMP 12.17	14.1	9.1	10,760	11S 379955E 4047534N	Large site under lodgepole pine forest
CAMP 12.18	15.2	8.0	11,150	11S 381333E 4047621N	Small site to the edge of willows as the trail climbs above Timberline Lake
CAMP 12.19	16.1	7.1	11,550	11S 382274E 4048125N	Many exposed, sandy sites among slabs and boulders on bluffs above the west end of Guitar Lake; beautiful views to the Kaweahs and Mt. Whitney; you must leave the trail to find these sites
CAMP 12.20	16.2	7.0	11,515	11S 382494E 4048041N	Many exposed, sandy sites among slabs between the trail and Guitar Lake; alpine scenery and beautiful views to Mt. Whitney

Camp ID	N–S	S–N	Elevation	UTM Coordinates (NAD27)	Description
CAMP 12.21	17.2	6.0	11,940	11S 383452E 4047401N	Many sites among slabs to the northern side of tarns; excellent views in all directions; you must leave the trail to find these sites
CAMP 12.22	19.0	4.2	13,320	11S 384294E 4046769N	Small, very exposed site at the end of the second-to-last switchback before the Whitney Trail junction
CAMP 12.23	19.1	4.1	13,380	11S 384351E 4046792N	Several small, very exposed, sandy sites among talus; upslope of the last switchback before the Whitney Trail junction
CAMP 12.24	19.3	3.9	13,560	11S 384430E 4046873N	Several small, very exposed, sandy sites among talus; just below the Sierra Crest; leave the Whitney Trail just north of the junction
CAMP 13.01	2.3	5.9	12,040	11S 385618E 4046947N	Trail Camp; many sites in sandy flats among slabs, on both sides of trail
CAMP 13.02	3.2	5.0	11,480	11S 386656E 4047421N	Small, sandy sites among slabs on open knob
CAMP 13.03	3.6	4.6	11,040	11S 387124E 4047496N	Medium-sized site beneath sparse tree cover; excellent views, but far from water
CAMP 13.04	3.9	4.3	10,860	11S 387145E 4047628N	Medium-sized site beneath foxtail pines; lovely site, but far from water
CAMP 13.05	4.6	3.6	10,370	11S 387453E 4047897N	Outpost Camp; large camping area beneath foxtail pines to the southwest of the creek crossing
CAMP 13.06	5.7	2.5	9990	11S 388234E 4048294N	Sites at Lone Pine Lake

APPENDIX D.

Bear Boxes

Location	N-S	S-N	Elevation	UTM Coordinates (NAD27)
Little Yosemite Valley (CAMP 1.01)	4.4	13.9	6130	11S 278409E 4179015N
Sunrise High Sierra Camp (CAMP 1.17)	13.1	5.2	9310	11S 285790E 4185522N
South side of Woods Creek crossing (CAMP 10.06)	7.3	8.6	8530	11S 371951E 4081607N
Arrowhead Lake (CAMP 10.10)	11.6	4.3	10,300	11S 374349E 4076467N
Northern Rae Lakes (CAMP 10.12)	12.6	3.3	10,560	11S 374736E 4075047N
Southern Rae Lakes (CAMP 10.14)	13.4	2.5	10,560	11S 375243E 4074150N
Charlotte Lakes* (CAMP 11.02)	2.3	9.5	10,400	11S 372816E 4070866N
Vidette Meadow (CAMP 11.09)	4.5	7.3	9550	11S 374559E 4068890N
Upper Vidette Meadow (CAMP 11.11)	5.3	6.5	9945	11S 375571E 4068228N
Center Basin junction (CAMP 11.15)	7.2	4.6	10,500	11S 377263E 4066001N
Tyndall Creek crossing (CAMP 12.02)	4.5	18.7	10,965	11S 376038E 4055964N
Tyndall Frog Ponds (CAMP 12.04)	5.4	17.8	11,025	11S 376211E 4055106N
Wallace Creek Crossing (CAMP 12.09)	9.3	13.9	10,400	11S 377465E 4050482N
Crabtree Meadow (CAMP 12.15)	13.6	9.6	10,700	11S 379335E 4047145N

* The Charlotte Lake bear box and campsite are 1 mile off the JMT at the northern end of Charlotte Lake.

Locations of bear boxes not on the JMT are available online at www.climber.org/data/Bear boxes.html.

APPENDIX E.

Side Trips to Peaks

More than 100 named summits lie within 2 miles of the John Muir Trail, and many have non-technical ascent routes. Described here are just 17 of them, chosen for their views, the straightforward route-finding to their summits, and, in many cases, for the absence of large amounts of loose talus. Few of the peaks described in this section are the tallest or most prominent in an area, but don't feel short-changed. The best views of a basin are usually from the slightly shorter peaks that lie in the middle of basins, rather than the tallest peaks that grace the crest.

If you plan to bag many summits while hiking the JMT, I recommend that you bring along a more exhaustive reference, such R.J. Secor's *High Sierra Peak, Passes, and Trails* (The Mountaineers Books, 1999) or Steve Roper's *The Climber's Guide to the High Sierra* (Sierra Club Books, 1976). However, if your schedule will allow just an occasional free afternoon to climb a peak, this selection is more than sufficient.

Section 1

Half Dome

Elevation: 8836 feet
Elevation Gain/Loss: ±1800 feet
Round-Trip Distance: 4 miles
Round-Trip Time: 4 hours

Climbing Half Dome has become nearly as much of a John Muir Trail requirement as summiting Mt. Whitney. Hide your pack at the Half Dome Trail junction, and proceed up the Half Dome Trail. The first mile and a bit are through forest, before you emerge on the granite slabs of Half Dome. The trail that ascends the first section of slabs is remarkable—the switchbacks are so well-constructed that you focus only on the steep steps, not the underlying slabs. A short descent brings you to Half Dome's famous cables. Take a breather, grab a pair of gloves, and proceed upward. Comfortingly, as with all domes, the slope lessens the higher you get, and the way down is much easier than you expect it to be. Enjoy the view down into Yosemite Valley and to the Yosemite high country.

Clouds Rest

Elevation: 9926 feet
Elevation Gain/Loss: ±2500 feet
Round-Trip Distance: 5 miles
Round-Trip Time: 5 hours

The north face of Clouds Rest is a nearly 5000-foot granite slab rising above Tenaya Canyon. While this peak is much less popular than Half Dome, its extra 1000 feet of elevation provide hikers with an even more stunning view of the Yosemite high country, as well as an excellent view of Half Dome. From the Clouds Rest junction, a half mile east of the Half Dome junction, head north up the Clouds Rest Trail. The summit is 2.5 miles and 2500 feet beyond this junction. Approximately a half mile before the summit is a trail junction: Be sure to take the left fork heading northeast to the summit of Clouds Rest. The right fork provides a route to Sunrise Lakes that circumvents Clouds Rest.

Columbia Finger

Elevation: 10,360 feet
Elevation Gain/Loss: ±800 feet
Round-Trip Distance: 1.8 miles
Round-Trip Time: 2-3 hours

Columbia Finger is the only technical peak included on this list, with a section of Class 3 climbing near the summit. Class 3 indicates that you will need to use handholds to ascend, but should never encounter terrain where you can fall more than 20 feet. If you find yourself on a section with more exposure, look around for an easier route or turn around. In Long Meadow, continue cross-country upstream where the John Muir Trail bends eastward. Once you are north of the summit of Columbia Finger, ascend the increasingly steep slabs and blocks northwest of the summit. For the final 100 to 200 feet, ascend blocks

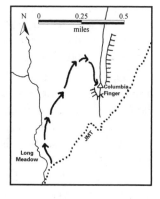

to the summit. The easiest route begins north of the summit and curves slowly to the southeast as you ascend. From the summit, enjoy the view north to Tresidder Peak, east to Matthes Crest—an impressively steep, milelong fin of rock—and south down Long Meadow and toward the Clark Range.

Section 2

Lembert Dome

Elevation: 9450 feet
Elevation Gain/Loss: ±800 feet
Round-Trip Distance: 2.8 miles
Round-Trip Time: 2-3 hours

Lembert Dome is a popular walk for all hikers visiting Tuolumne Meadows. The hike begins at a parking lot along the Tuolumne Lodge road, 0.4 mile east of the wilderness permit office. The trail climbs north through forest for 0.5 mile to a junction. Head left to reach Lembert Dome. After 0.4 mile, the trail reaches the saddle between the two summits and vanishes. From here, follow slabs south to the summit. Lembert Dome is an excellent vantage point for the Tuolumne Meadows area, with views of Mt. Dana and Mt. Gibbs to the east, Lyell Canyon to the south, and the Cathedral Range and Tuolumne Meadows to the west. (On your return trip, you can either retrace your steps at the trail junction east of the summit, or continue north. The trail loops north around Lembert Dome, ending at the Lembert Dome parking area.)

Donohue Peak

Elevation: 12,023 feet
Elevation Gain/Loss: ±1300 feet
Round-Trip Distance: 3.3 miles
Round-Trip Time: 3 hours

Donohue Peak is a bit of a talus slog, but with an excellent view down Lyell Canyon and south into the San Joaquin drainage. From Donohue Pass, head cross-country north either up and over Peak 11,263, or skirt around its western edge. From the lake north of Peak 11,263, head northeast either up the ridge or just to the left of the ridge to the summit of Donohue Peak. Although this route is mostly talus, the talus is quite stable. The first ascent of the peak was made on horseback from the northwest.

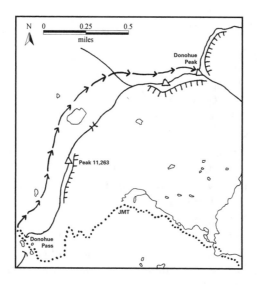

Section 4

Red Cones

Elevation: 9032 feet
Elevation Gain/Loss: ±400 feet
Round-Trip Distance: 0.5 mile
Round-Trip Time: Less than 1 hour

The Red Cones are a pair of cinder cones on either side of the Crater Creek crossing, which is just north of Crater Meadow. Both sport excellent views of the Ritter Range and the John Muir Trail as far north as Donohue Pass. While the northern, and shorter, cone, is less vegetated near the summit, I prefer the view from the southern, taller cone. From the creek crossing, head cross-country and ascend the northern cone anywhere along its southwestern flank; you will undoubtedly find use trails in the unstable cinders. The southern cone can be ascended anywhere along its eastern or northeastern sides, but a less direct and less steep route allows you to minimize the frustration of "two steps climbed up, one step slid back down." The best vista points are slightly west of the summit.

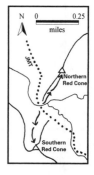

Section 6

Volcanic Knob

Elevation: 11,140 feet
Elevation Gain/Loss: ±1400 feet
Round-Trip Distance: 3.5 miles
Round-Trip Time: 4-5 hours

Volcanic Knob requires a bit more of a detour and more complex route-finding than most peaks listed, but it is well worth the walk past two hidden meadows to a phenomenal vista point. This peak should not be attempted unless you are carrying a compass or GPS, as the peak is not visible from where you leave the JMT. To reach Volcanic Knob, leave the JMT at the Bear Ridge Trail junction. Head cross-country up a small gully, trending northwest toward the southern edges of the two meadows. In the first, you will find a snow survey cabin and automated weather station. Heading east-northeast, pass over the small ridge to the second meadow and begin your climb of Volcanic Knob. The walking is easiest if you trend a bit south, to the right side of the peak, staying in the trees. Taking this route, you will encounter no talus. From the summit, you have a view northward of the Silver Divide and Silver Pass, to the west of Lake Thomas Edison, and to the south to Recess Peak, Seven Gables, and Selden Pass.

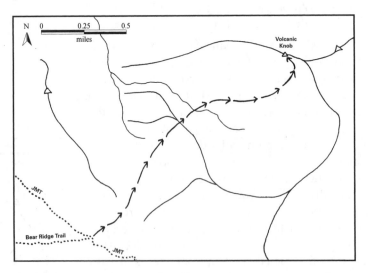

Section 7

Mt. Spencer

Elevation: 12,431 feet
Elevation Gain/Loss: ±1500 feet
Round-Trip Distance: 2.5 miles
Round-Trip Time: 3-4 hours

Mt. Spencer is the lowest of the peaks in Evolution Basin, but its central position means you have excellent views in all directions, especially of the west faces of Mt. Darwin and Mt. Mendel. From the southern section of the eastern shore of Sapphire Lake (the easiest way to reach the eastern shore of Sapphire Lake is to leave the John Muir Trail at Sapphire Lake's outlet), head cross-country up the southwesterly spur extending from Mt. Spencer. This spur leads to southern end of Mt. Spencer's summit ridge (at approximately 12,200 feet). From here, head north along the west side of the ridge on slabs, blocks, and sandy patches amongst the rocky outcrops.

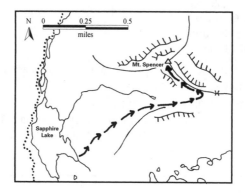

Mt. Solomons

Elevation: 13,034 feet
Elevation Gain/Loss: ±1100 feet
Round-Trip Distance: 1.2 miles
Round-Trip Time: 2-3 hours

Mt. Solomons provides a glance into the Ionian Basin, just southwest of Muir Pass, and an especially good view of Charybdis, one of the two peaks guarding the start of the Enchanted Gorge. Mt. Solomons has also long been a favorite of mine, as it is named after Theodore Solomons, the man who first proposed the construction of the John Muir

Trail and named many of the peaks in Evolution Basin. To ascend Mt. Solomons, first head south-southwest cross-country up the slope from Muir Pass. After approximately 200 feet of elevation gain, contour westward for approximately 0.15 mile to avoid the cliffs straight ahead. Then resume climbing up the northwest rib on talus. Be careful, as some rocks will be loose. Once on the summit ridge, head east to the high point. The peak due south of you, sporting a giant rockslide on its northern face, is Charybdis.

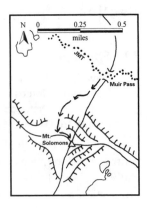

Section 8

Black Giant

Elevation: 13,330 feet
Elevation Gain/Loss: ±1600 feet
Round-Trip Distance: 3 miles
Round-Trip Time: 4-5 hours

Since it is tall, yet stands apart from other tall peaks along the Sierra Crest, the view from the Black Giant is rather overwhelming—to the south is a seemingly endless sea of peaks and valleys all the way to Mt. Whitney and the Kaweahs. Remarkably, there is a Class 1 route up the Black Giant, indicating easy walking with minimal talus. Just above the

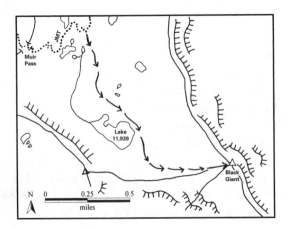

highest Helen Lake inlet, head south cross-country to not-yet-visible Lake 11,939. The landscape is full of small lumps; always aim for the lowest of them to avoid unnecessary elevation loss as you approach the lake. Skirt Lake 11,939 along its northern and eastern shores, heading for the shallow pass to its south. Just before you reach the pass, begin ascending the far southern section of the Black Giant's western slope; the easiest walking is where a slight ridge is visible. Trending due east brings you to the summit. Afternoon lighting is best, and be sure to leave yourself ample time to just sit and gaze at the views.

Section 9

Split Mountain

Elevation: 14,042 feet
Elevation Gain/Loss: ±2400 feet
Round-Trip Distance: 5 miles
Round-Trip Time: 6-7 hours

Besides Mt. Whitney, Split Mountain is the easiest 14,000-foot peak you will pass on the John Muir Trail. From the northern end of Upper Basin, head due east cross-country to Lake 11,595 (3535 meters). Head around the southern side of the lake and up easy slopes, to the side of the drainage, toward the Sierra Crest. Once you are at approximately 12,400 feet, you will note the long, gentle, easy talus slope heading south to the summit of Split Mountain. Ascend it to enjoy a view eastward to the Inyo and White mountains, and the Owens Valley and expansive views of the Sierra in all other directions.

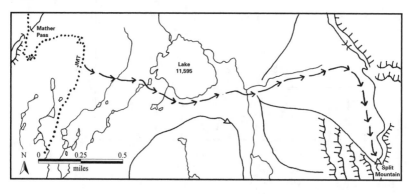

Section 10

Crater Mountain

Elevation: 12,874 feet
Elevation Gain/Loss: ±1400 feet
Round-Trip Distance: 2 miles
Round-Trip Time: 3-4 hours

The summit of Crater Mountain has open vistas to Mt. Clarence King in the south and the White Fork of Woods Creek to the west. While there is loose, metamorphic rock near the summit of the peak, the going is much easier than on nearby summits, including Mt. Pinchot, Mt. Perkins, and Mt. Ickes. From approximately 11,500 feet on the south side of Pinchot Pass, head cross-country up the northeastern spur of Crater Mountain; the rock is much more stable than in the bowl to the north. Just before the summit, the terrain becomes steeper, and you must head a short distance west on a narrow ridge to reach high point. The view from Crater Mountain is much better than it is from Pinchot Pass. You are farther west, and the massive ridge southwest of Sawmill Pass no longer obstructs your view toward Mt. Clarence King, the steep pyramid just south of Woods Creek.

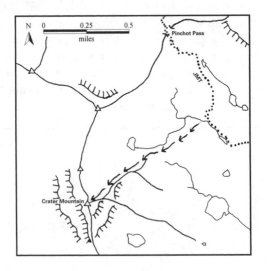

Painted Lady

Elevation: 12,119 feet
Elevation Gain/Loss: ±750 feet
Round-Trip Distance: 1.2 miles
Round-Trip Time: 2 hours

If you are willing to put up with a 500-foot ascent on loose talus, you will be rewarded with a fantastic view of the Rae Lakes from the summit of the Painted Lady. Just 500 feet down the north side of Glen Pass is a flat, talus-laden basin dotted with small tarns. Head east cross-country from this point to the Painted Lady, a large pile of colorful metamorphic talus. Climb along the west spur toward the steeper talus that ascends the final 500 feet to the summit. You will encounter somewhat more stable rock if you stick a little south of the west rib. From the summit, enjoy the view east to Dragon Peak and north to the Rae Lakes.

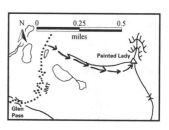

Section 11

Mt. Bago

Elevation: 11,870 feet
Elevation Gain/Loss: ±1850 feet from JMT
Round-Trip Distance: 2 miles from Charlotte Lake inlet;
    3.3 miles from JMT junction
Round-Trip Time: 4 hours from JMT

Mt. Bago stands alone at the head of Bubbs Creek, with views to Charlotte Dome to the west and the Great Western and Kings-Kern divides to the south. From the Charlotte Lake inlet, head due west cross-country up the forested slope to the lower, eastern summit of Mt. Bago. There is a short stretch of loose gravel just below the ridgeline. Follow the nearly flat ridge south to the higher summit. The pyramid-shaped peak to the southwest is Mt. Brewer, flanked on either side by South Guard and North Guard. Due south is the very rugged Kings-Kern

Divide. Most of the peaks along it have only technical ascent routes, and the passes are equally steep to cross.

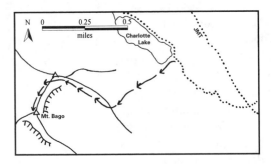

Section 12

Caltech Peak

Elevation: 13,832 feet
Elevation Gain/Loss: ±1800 feet
Round-Trip Distance: 2 miles
Round-Trip Time: 3-4 hours

An ascent of Caltech Peak will provide you with a vista to the Lake South America Basin, the Great Western Divide, and the JMT south of Forester Pass. From the JMT, there are many possible routes to the summit of Caltech Peak. The farther south you ascend the summit ridge, the less steep the route, but it is longer. I recommend that you leave the JMT near the outlet of the second large lake south of Forester Pass, at an approximate

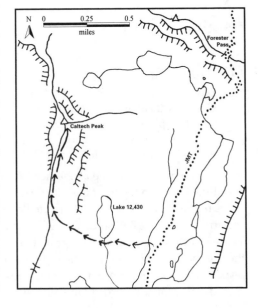

elevation of 12,070 feet. Head west across the outlet of Lake 12,430 feet (3780+ meters) and ascend toward the northwest to the ridge south of Caltech Peak. You will encounter talus on the steeper sections of this climb. From the ridge, you traverse relatively easy talus north to the summit. To the west, you are looking at the southern Great Western Divide. From south to north, Milestone (the pinnacle), Midday Mountain (the nondescript peak), Table Mountain (the flat-topped peak), and Thunder Mountain (the steep pyramid) dominate the view.

Tawny Point

> **Elevation:** 12,332 feet
> **Elevation Gain/Loss:** ±900 feet
> **Round-Trip Distance:** 1.5 miles
> **Round-Trip Time:** 2 hours

Tawny Point is an easy hike from Bighorn Plateau, with exquisite views of the entire Kern Basin. If you climb just one peak while hiking the John Muir Trail, this is my recommendation. From the Tyndall Creek crossing south to the western Crabtree junction, you are walking along a shelf to the east of the Kern River. The view from Tawny Point provides a vista into the remarkably straight Kern drainage, west to the rugged peaks of the Kaweahs and the Great Western Divide, north to the upper Kern along the Kings-Kern Divide, and southeast to the Mt. Whitney area. From Bighorn Plateau, head slightly northeast cross-country and then north up the southern slope of Tawny Point. There are no routefinding obstacles or talus en route to the summit.

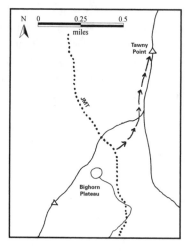

Section 13

Wotans Throne

Elevation: 12,726 feet
Elevation Gain: ±700 feet
Round-Trip Distance: 1 mile
Round-Trip Time: 2 hours

Wotans Throne has a superb view of the east face of Mt. Whitney, especially at sunrise. If you have just hiked the trail north to south and are camped at Trail Camp, this is a worthwhile detour before heading down to Whitney Portal on your last morning. From Trail Camp, head north cross-country up the right side of drainage from the small lake, staying left of the steep slabs. Where the slope of the drainage lessens, head west (left) onto the crest of the rock glacier—despite the deceptive appearance from below, this will lead you to easy walking terrain. Continue north until you are at the northwest corner of the peak. Ascend slabs and talus at either the northwest corner or the northern face to reach the summit. Avoid the temptation to start ascending too early, or you will encounter much steeper terrain.

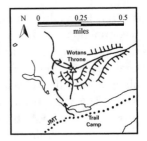

APPENDIX F.

Topographic Maps

The maps included in this book are derived from *The John Muir Trail Map-Pack* published by Tom Harrison. While the maps here suffice for planning purposes, most hikers will wish to have more detail for the hike itself in order to explore areas off the JMT or to gain a better understanding of the surrounding terrain.

The following sheet maps are popular options for JMT hikers:

The John Muir Trail Map-Pack is a collection of 13 full-color, 8.5 x 11 sheets, covering the length of the trail (www.tomharrisonmaps.com). Scale 1:63360.

The High Country series provides more detail for the routes to and from the JMT with the following maps: *Yosemite High Country, Mammoth High Country, Mono Divide High Country, Kings Canyon High Country,* and *Mt. Whitney High Country* (www.tomharrisonmaps.com). Scale 1: 63360.

The USGS 7.5-minute topographic maps can be ordered directly from USGS (store.usgs.gov); some are available in a limited number of stores. Note that not all are up to date or accurate regarding the current JMT route. The following USGS 7.5-minute maps cover the entire JMT. Abbreviations like "Mtn." reflect the actual name used on the topo. Additional 7.5-minute maps needed to cover routes to and from the JMT are listed in Appendix B.

Half Dome	*Bloody Mtn.*	*Split Mtn.*
Merced Peak	*Graveyard Peak*	*Mt. Pinchot*
Tenaya Lake	*Florence Lake*	*Mt. Clarence King*
Vogelsang Peak	*Mt. Hilgard*	*Mt. Williamson*
Tioga Pass	*Ward Mountain*	*Mt. Brewer*
Koip Peak	*Mt. Henry*	*Mt. Kaweah*
Mt. Ritter	*Mt. Darwin*	*Mt. Whitney*
Mammoth Mtn.	*Mt. Goddard*	
Crystal Crag	*North Palisade*	

APPENDIX G.

Plants Referenced in Text

Plant names referenced in text, indexed by common name

Common Name	Scientific Name	Family
Agoseris, short-beaked	*Agoseris glauca*	Asteraceae
Alpine gold	*Hulsea algida*	Asteraceae
Alpineflames	*Pyrrocoma apargioides*	Asteraceae
Angelica, Sierra	*Angelica lineariloba*	Apiaceae
Arnica, Sierra	*Arnica nevadensis*	Asteraceae
Aspen, quaking	*Populus tremuloides*	Salicaceae
Aster, alpine	*Aster alpigenus*	Asteraceae
Azalea, western	*Rhododendron occidentalis*	Ericaceae
Bay-laurel, California	*Umbellularia californica*	Lauraceae
Beardtongue, Rothrock's	*Keckiella rothrockii*	Scrophulariaceae
Bilberry, dwarf	*Vaccinium caespitosum*	Ericaceae
Bistort, western	*Polygonum bistortoides*	Polygonaceae
Blueberry, western	*Vaccinium uliginosum*	Ericaceae
Buckwheat, foxtail	*Eriogonum polypodum*	Polygonaceae
Buckwheat, frosted	*Eriogonum incanum*	Polygonaceae
Buckwheat, oval-leaved	*Eriogonum ovalifolium*	Polygonaceae
Bush chinquapin	*Chrysolepis sempervirens*	Fagaceae
Buttercup, Eschscholtz'	*Ranunculus eschscholtzii*	Ranunculaceae
Cinquefoil, Bush	*Potentilla fruticosa*	Rosaceae
Cliff bush	*Jamesia americana*	Philadelphaceae
Clover, carpet	*Trifolium monanthum*	Fabaceae
Columbine, crimson	*Aquilegia formosa*	Ranunculaceae
Cream bush, small-leaved	*Holodiscus microphyllus*	Rosaceae
Currant, alpine prickly	*Ribes montigenum*	Grossulariaceae
Currant, wax	*Ribes cereum*	Grossulariaceae
Daisy, Coulter's	*Erigeron coulteri*	Asteraceae
Daisy, Sierra cutleaf	*Erigeron compositus*	Asteraceae
Daisy, Sierra fleabane	*Erigeron aldigus*	Asteraceae
Douglas fir	*Pseudotsuga menziesii*	Pinaceae
Draba, granite	*Draba lemmonii*	Brassicaceae
Elderberry, mountain red	*Sambucus racemosa*	Caprifoliaceae
Elephant's head, little	*Pedicularis attolens*	Scrophulariaceae
Eupatorium, western	*Ageratina occidentalis*	Asteraceae
Fernbush	*Chamaebatiaria millefolium*	Rosaceae
Fir, red	*Abies magnificata*	Pinaceae
Fir, white	*Abies concolor*	Pinaceae

Common Name	Scientific Name	Family
Fireweed	*Epilobium angustifolium*	Onagraceae
Flax, western blue	*Linum lewisii*	Linaceae
Fuchsia, California	*Epilobium canum*	Onagraceae
Gentian, alpine	*Gentiana newberryi*	Gentianaceae
Gentian, perennial	*Swertia perennis*	Gentianaceae
Gentian, Sierra	*Gentianopsis holopetala*	Gentianaceae
Goldenrod, alpine	*Solidago multiradiata*	Asteraceae
Gooseberry, Sierra	*Ribes roezlii*	Grossulariaceae
Granite gilia	*Leptodactylon pungens*	Polemoniaceae
Grass-of-Parnassus	*Parnassia californica*	Saxifragaceae
Groundsel, arrow-leaved	*Senecio triangularis*	Asteraceae
Groundsel, Fremont's	*Senecio fremontii*	Asteraceae
Hawkweed, shaggy	*Hieracium horridum*	Asteraceae
Heather, red mountain	*Phyllodoce breweri*	Ericaceae
Heather, white mountain	*Cassiope mertensiana*	Ericaceae
Hemlock, mountain	*Tsuga mertensiana*	Pinaceae
Heuchera, pink	*Heuchera rubescens*	Saxifragaceae
Incense cedar	*Calocedrus decurrens*	Cupressaceae
Ivesia, club-moss	*Ivesia lycopodioides*	Rosaceae
Ivesia, mousetail	*Ivesia santolinoides*	Rosaceae
Ivesia, Muir's	*Ivesia muirii*	Rosaceae
Juniper, western	*Juniperus occidentalis*	Cupressaceae
Kalmia, bog	*Kalmia polifolia*	Ericaceae
Labrador tea, western	*Ledum glandulosum*	Ericaceae
Lily, corn	*Veratrum californicum*	Liliaceae
Lily, Kelley's tiger	*Lilium kelleyanum*	Liliaceae
Manzanita, greenleaf	*Arctostaphylos patula*	Ericaceae
Manzanita, pinemat	*Arctostaphylos nevadensis*	Ericaceae
Maple, big-leaf	*Acer macrophyllum*	Aceraceae
Mariposa lily, Leichtlin's	*Calochortus leichtlinii*	Liliaceae
Monkeyflower, mountain	*Mimulus tilingii*	Scrophulariaceae
Monkeyflower, primrose	*Mimulus primuloides*	Scrophulariaceae
Mountain mahogany	*Cercocarpus ledifolius*	Rosaceae
Oak, California black	*Quercus kelloggii*	Fagaceae
Oak, canyon live	*Quercus chrysolepis*	Fagaceae
Onion, swamp	*Allium validum*	Liliaceae
Orchid, Sierra rein	*Platanthera leucostachys*	Orchidaceae
Paintbrush, alpine	*Castilleja nana*	Scrophulariaceae
Paintbrush, great red	*Castilleja miniata*	Scrophulariaceae
Paintbrush, Lemmon's	*Castilleja lemmonii*	Scrophulariaceae
Paintbrush, mountain	*Castilleja parviflora*	Scrophulariaceae
Paintbrush, wavy-leaved	*Castilleja applegatei*	Scrophulariaceae
Pennyroyal	*Monardella odoratissima*	Lamiaceae
Penstemon, mountain pride	*Penstemon newberryi*	Scrophulariaceae
Penstemon, scarlet	*Penstemon rostriflorus*	Scrophulariaceae
Penstemon, showy	*Penstemon speciosus*	Scrophulariaceae
Penstemon, Sierra	*Penstemon heterodoxus*	Scrophulariaceae

Common Name	Scientific Name	Family
Phlox, spreading	*Phlox diffusa*	Polemoniaceae
Pine, foxtail	*Pinus balfouriana*	Pinaceae
Pine, Jeffrey	*Pinus jeffreyi*	Pinaceae
Pine, lodgepole	*Pinus contorta*	Pinaceae
Pine, single-leaf pinyon	*Pinus monophylla*	Pinaceae
Pine, sugar	*Pinus lambertiana*	Pinaceae
Pine, western white	*Pinus monticola*	Pinaceae
Pine, whitebark	*Pinus albicaulis*	Pinaceae
Pretty faces	*Triteleia ixioides*	Liliaceae
Primrose, Sierra	*Primula suffretescens*	Primulaceae
Pussypaws	*Calyptridium umbellatum*	Portulacaceae
Pussytoes, flat-topped	*Antennaria corymbosa*	Asteraceae
Pussytoes, rosy	*Antennaria rosea*	Asteraceae
Ranger's buttons	*Sphenosciadium capitellatum*	Apiaceae
Rock cress	*Arabis sp.*	Brassicaceae
Rockfringe	*Epilobium obcordatum*	Onagraceae
Sagebrush, mountain	*Artemisia tridentata*	Asteraceae
Sandwort, Nuttall's	*Minuartia nuttallii*	Caryophyllaceae
Saxifrage, bud	*Saxifraga bryophora*	Saxifragaceae
Sedge	*Carex sp.*	Cyperaceae
Sedum, rosy	*Sedum rosea*	Crassulaceae
Shooting star, mountaineer	*Dodecatheon redolens*	Primulaceae
Silktassel, Fremont	*Garrya fremontii*	Garryaceae
Sky pilot	*Polemonium eximium*	Polemoniaceae
Sneezeweed, Bigelow's	*Helenium bigelovii*	Asteraceae
Sneezeweed, orange	*Dugaldia hoopesii*	Asteraceae
Snow plant	*Sarcodes sanguinea*	Ericaceae
Snowberry, creeping	*Symphoricarpos mollis*	Caprifoliaceae
Sorrel, mountain	*Oxyria digyna*	Polygonaceae
Spiraea, dense-flowered	*Spiraea densiflora*	Rosaceae
Stonecrop, Sierra	*Sedum obtusatum*	Crassulaceae
Thistle, Anderson's	*Cirsium andersonii*	Asteraceae
Thistle, elk	*Cirsium scariosum*	Asteraceae
Wallflower, western	*Erysimum capitatum*	Brassicaceae
Whitethorn, mountain	*Ceanothus cordulatus*	Rhamnaceae
Willow, arctic	*Salix arctica*	Salicaceae
Yampah, Parish's	*Perideridia parishii*	Apiaceae

Plant names referenced in text, indexed by scientific name
(alphabetized by family)

Common Name	Scientific Name	Family
Maple, big-leaf	*Acer macrophyllum*	Aceraceae
Angelica, Sierra	*Angelica lineariloba*	Apiaceae
Yampah, Parish's	*Perideridia parishii*	Apiaceae
Ranger's buttons	*Sphenosciadium capitellatum*	Apiaceae
Eupatorium, western	*Ageratina occidentalis*	Asteraceae
Agoseris, short-beaked	*Agoseris glauca*	Asteraceae
Pussytoes, flat-topped	*Antennaria corymbosa*	Asteraceae
Pussytoes, rosy	*Antennaria rosea*	Asteraceae
Arnica, Sierra	*Arnica nevadensis*	Asteraceae
Sagebrush, mountain	*Artemisia tridentata*	Asteraceae
Aster, alpine	*Aster alpigenus*	Asteraceae
Thistle, Anderson's	*Cirsium andersonii*	Asteraceae
Thistle, elk	*Cirsium scariosum*	Asteraceae
Sneezeweed, orange	*Dugaldia hoopesii*	Asteraceae
Daisy, Sierra fleabane	*Erigeron aldigus*	Asteraceae
Daisy, Sierra cutleaf	*Erigeron compositus*	Asteraceae
Daisy, Coulter's	*Erigeron coulteri*	Asteraceae
Sneezeweed, Bigelow's	*Helenium bigelovii*	Asteraceae
Hawkweed, shaggy	*Hieracium horridum*	Asteraceae
Alpine gold	*Hulsea algida*	Asteraceae
Alpineflames	*Pyrrocoma apargioides*	Asteraceae
Groundsel, Fremont's	*Senecio fremontii*	Asteraceae
Groundsel, arrow-leaved	*Senecio triangularis*	Asteraceae
Goldenrod, alpine	*Solidago multiradiata*	Asteraceae
Rock cress	*Arabis sp.*	Brassicaceae
Draba, granite	*Draba lemmonii*	Brassicaceae
Wallflower, western	*Erysimum capitatum*	Brassicaceae
Elderberry, mountain red	*Sambucus racemosa*	Caprifoliaceae
Snowberry, creeping	*Symphoricarpos mollis*	Caprifoliaceae
Sandwort, Nuttall's	*Minuartia nuttallii*	Caryophyllaceae
Stonecrop, Sierra	*Sedum obtusatum*	Crassulaceae
Sedum, rosy	*Sedum rosea*	Crassulaceae
Incense cedar	*Calocedrus decurrens*	Cupressaceae
Juniper, western	*Juniperus occidentalis*	Cupressaceae
Sedge	*Carex sp.*	Cyperaceae
Manzanita, pinemat	*Arctostaphylos nevadensis*	Ericaceae
Manzanita, greenleaf	*Arctostaphylos patula*	Ericaceae
Heather, white mountain	*Cassiope mertensiana*	Ericaceae
Kalmia, bog	*Kalmia polifolia*	Ericaceae
Labrador tea, western	*Ledum glandulosum*	Ericaceae
Heather, red mountain	*Phyllodoce breweri*	Ericaceae
Azalea, western	*Rhododendron occidentalis*	Ericaceae
Snow plant	*Sarcodes sanguinea*	Ericaceae
Bilberry, dwarf	*Vaccinium caespitosum*	Ericaceae

Common Name	Scientific Name	Family
Blueberry, western	*Vaccinium uliginosum*	Ericaceae
Clover, carpet	*Trifolium monanthum*	Fabaceae
Bush chinquapin	*Chrysolepis sempervirens*	Fagaceae
Oak, canyon live	*Quercus chrysolepis*	Fagaceae
Oak, California black	*Quercus kelloggii*	Fagaceae
Silktassel, Fremont	*Garrya fremontii*	Garryaceae
Gentian, alpine	*Gentiana newberryi*	Gentianaceae
Gentian, Sierra	*Gentianopsis holopetala*	Gentianaceae
Gentian, perennial	*Swertia perennis*	Gentianaceae
Currant, wax	*Ribes cereum*	Grossulariaceae
Currant, alpine prickly	*Ribes montigenum*	Grossulariaceae
Gooseberry, Sierra	*Ribes roezlii*	Grossulariaceae
Pennyroyal	*Monardella odoratissima*	Lamiaceae
Bay-laurel, California	*Umbellularia californica*	Lauraceae
Onion, swamp	*Allium validum*	Liliaceae
Mariposa lily, Leichtlin's	*Calochortus leichtlinii*	Liliaceae
Lily, Kelley's tiger	*Lilium kelleyanum*	Liliaceae
Pretty faces	*Triteleia ixioides*	Liliaceae
Lily, corn	*Veratrum californicum*	Liliaceae
Flax, western blue	*Linum lewisii*	Linaceae
Fireweed	*Epilobium angustifolium*	Onagraceae
Fuchsia, California	*Epilobium canum*	Onagraceae
Rockfringe	*Epilobium obcordatum*	Onagraceae
Orchid, Sierra rein	*Platanthera leucostachys*	Orchidaceae
Cliff bush	*Jamesia americana*	Philadelphaceae
Fir, white	*Abies concolor*	Pinaceae
Fir, red	*Abies magnificata*	Pinaceae
Pine, whitebark	*Pinus albicaulis*	Pinaceae
Pine, foxtail	*Pinus balfouriana*	Pinaceae
Pine, lodgepole	*Pinus contorta*	Pinaceae
Pine, Jeffrey	*Pinus jeffreyi*	Pinaceae
Pine, sugar	*Pinus lambertiana*	Pinaceae
Pine, single-leaf pinyon	*Pinus monophylla*	Pinaceae
Pine, western white	*Pinus monticola*	Pinaceae
Douglas fir	*Pseudotsuga menziesii*	Pinaceae
Hemlock, mountain	*Tsuga mertensiana*	Pinaceae
Granite gilia	*Leptodactylon pungens*	Polemoniaceae
Phlox, spreading	*Phlox diffusa*	Polemoniaceae
Sky pilot	*Polemonium eximium*	Polemoniaceae
Buckwheat, frosted	*Eriogonum incanum*	Polygonaceae
Buckwheat, oval-leaved	*Eriogonum ovalifolium*	Polygonaceae
Buckwheat, foxtail	*Eriogonum polypodum*	Polygonaceae
Sorrel, mountain	*Oxyria digyna*	Polygonaceae
Bistort, western	*Polygonum bistortoides*	Polygonaceae
Pussypaws	*Calyptridium umbellatum*	Portulacaceae
Shooting star, mountaineer	*Dodecatheon redolens*	Primulaceae
Primrose, Sierra	*Primula suffretescens*	Primulaceae

Common Name	Scientific Name	Family
Columbine, crimson	*Aquilegia formosa*	Ranunculaceae
Buttercup, Eschscholtz'	*Ranunculus eschscholtzii*	Ranunculaceae
Whitethorn, mountain	*Ceanothus cordulatus*	Rhamnaceae
Mountain mahogany	*Cercocarpus ledifolius*	Rosaceae
Fernbush	*Chamaebatiaria millefolium*	Rosaceae
Cream bush, small-leaved	*Holodiscus microphyllus*	Rosaceae
Ivesia, Club-moss	*Ivesia lycopodioides*	Rosaceae
Ivesia, Muir's	*Ivesia muirii*	Rosaceae
Ivesia, mousetail	*Ivesia santolinoides*	Rosaceae
Cinquefoil, bush	*Potentilla fruticosa*	Rosaceae
Spiraea, dense-flowered	*Spiraea densiflora*	Rosaceae
Aspen, quaking	*Populus tremuloides*	Salicaceae
Willow, arctic	*Salix arctica*	Salicaceae
Heuchera, pink	*Heuchera rubescens*	Saxifragaceae
Grass-of-Parnassus	*Parnassia californica*	Saxifragaceae
Saxifrage, bud	*Saxifraga bryophora*	Saxifragaceae
Paintbrush, wavy-leaved	*Castilleja applegatei*	Scrophulariaceae
Paintbrush, Lemmon's	*Castilleja lemmonii*	Scrophulariaceae
Paintbrush, great red	*Castilleja miniata*	Scrophulariaceae
Paintbrush, alpine	*Castilleja nana*	Scrophulariaceae
Paintbrush, mountain	*Castilleja parviflora*	Scrophulariaceae
Beardtongue, Rothrock's	*Keckiella rothrockii*	Scrophulariaceae
Monkeyflower, primrose	*Mimulus primuloides*	Scrophulariaceae
Monkeyflower, mountain	*Mimulus tilingii*	Scrophulariaceae
Elephant's head, little	*Pedicularis attolens*	Scrophulariaceae
Penstemon, Sierra	*Penstemon heterodoxus*	Scrophulariaceae
Penstemon, mountain pride	*Penstemon newberryi*	Scrophulariaceae
Penstemon, scarlet	*Penstemon rostriflorus*	Scrophulariaceae
Penstemon, showy	*Penstemon speciosus*	Scrophulariaceae

APPENDIX H.

Bibliography and Suggested Reading

Beedy, E.C. *Discovering Sierra Birds: Western Slope*. El Portal, CA: Yosemite Natural History Association and Sequoia Natural History Association, 1985.

Blackwell, L.R. *Wildflowers of the Sierra Nevada and the Central Valley*. Edmonton, Canada: Lone Pine Press, 1999.

Brewer, W. H., and W. H. Alsup. *Such a Landscape!: A Narrative of the 1864 California Geological Survey Exploration of Yosemite, Sequoia & Kings Canyon from the Diary, Field Notes, Letters & Reports of William Henry Brewer*. Yosemite National Park, CA: Yosemite Association, 1999.

Browning, P. *Place Names of the Sierra Nevada: From Abbot to Zumwalt*. Berkeley, CA: Wilderness Press, 1991 [out of print].

Farquhar, F. P. *History of the Sierra Nevada*. Berkeley, CA: University of California Press, 1965.

King, C. F. F. P. *Mountaineering in the Sierra Nevada*. Lincoln, NE: University of Nebraska Press, 1997.

Gaines, D. *Birds of Yosemite and the East Slope*. Lee Vining, CA: Artemisia Press, 1992.

Guyton, B. *Glaciers of California: Modern Glaciers, Ice Age Glaciers, Origin of Yosemite Valley, and a Glacier Tour in the Sierra Nevada*. Berkeley, CA: University of California Press, 1998.

Hill, M. *Geology of the Sierra Nevada*. Berkeley, CA: University of California Press, 2006.

Horn, E.L. *Sierra Nevada Wildflowers*. Missoula, MT: Mountain Press Publishing Company, 1998.

Huber, N.K., and W.W.C. Eckhardt. *The Story of Devils Postpile.* Three Rivers, CA: Sequoia Natural History Association, 2002.

Jameson, E.W., and H.J. Peeters. *Mammals of California.* Berkeley, CA: University of California Press, 2004.

Johnston, V.R. *Sierra Nevada: The Naturalist's Companion.* Berkeley, CA: University of California Press, 1998.

Moore, J.G. *Exploring the Highest Sierra.* Stanford, CA: Stanford University Press, 2000.

Roth, H. *Pathway in the Sky.* Berkeley, CA: Howell-North Books, 1965.

Sargent, S. *Solomons of the Sierra: The Pioneer of the John Muir Trail.* Yosemite, CA: Flying Spur Press, 1989.

Sibley, D.A., *The Sibley Field Guide to Birds of Western North America.* New York: Alfred A. Knopf, 2003.

Storer, T.I., R.L. Usinger, and D. Lukas. *Sierra Nevada Natural History.* Berkeley, CA: University of California Press, 2004.

Weeden, N. *A Sierra Nevada Flora.* Berkeley, CA: Wilderness Press, 1996.

INDEX

ABOUT THE AUTHORS

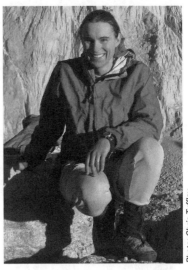

From childhood, **Lizzy Wenk** has hiked and climbed in the Sierra Nevada with her family. After she started college, she found excuses to spend every summer in the Sierra, with its beguiling landscape, abundant flowers, and near-perfect weather. During those summers, she worked as a research assistant for others and completed her own Ph.D. thesis research on the effects of rock type on alpine plant distribution and physiology. But much of the time, she hikes simply for leisure. Obsessively wanting to explore every bit of the Sierra, she has hiked thousands of on- and off-trail miles and climbed nearly 500 peaks in the mountain range. Since 2005, she and her husband, Douglas, have lived full time in Bishop, California. She teaches biology at Cerro Coso Community College, and most recently has been busy caring for her daughter, Eleanor.

Kathy Morey has authored and co-authored numerous books for Wilderness Press, including four hiking guides on Hawaii, *Hot Showers, Soft Beds, and Dayhikes in the Sierra*, *Sierra North*, and *Sierra South*. She lives in Big Pine, California.